Liver Transplantation - Challenges and Opportunities

Edited by Georgios Tsoulfas

Published in London, United Kingdom

Liver Transplantation - Challenges and Opportunities
http://dx.doi.org/10.5772/intechopen.111341
Edited by Georgios Tsoulfas

Contributors
Ahmed H. Abdelwahed, Bill S. Majdalany, Brian L. Shaw, Carlos E. Marroquin, Eleni Avramidou, Elizabeth Richardson, Georgios Tsoulfas, Jesus Bautista, Kristopher Croome, Nam Hoang Duc, Rohan M. Goswami, Shriya Sharma, Stella Vasileiadou

First published in London, United Kingdom, 2024 by IntechOpen
IntechOpen is the global imprint of INTECHOPEN LIMITED, registered in England and Wales, registration number: 11086078, 167-169 Great Portland Street, London, W1W 5PF, United Kingdom

British Library Cataloguing-in-Publication Data
A catalogue record for this book is available from the British Library

Additional hard and PDF copies can be obtained from orders@intechopen.com

Liver Transplantation - Challenges and Opportunities
Edited by Georgios Tsoulfas
p. cm.
Print ISBN 978-0-85466-035-3
Online ISBN 978-0-85466-034-6
eBook (PDF) ISBN 978-0-85466-036-0

For EU product safety concerns:
IN TECH d.o.o., Prolaz Marije Krucifikse Kozulić 3, 51000 Rijeka, Croatia,
info@intechopen.com or visit our website at intechopen.com.

Meet the editor

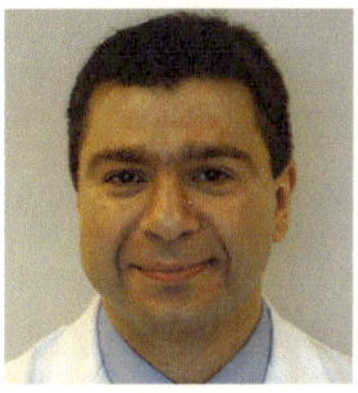

Dr. Georgios Tsoulfas received his MD from Brown University School of Medicine and completed a general surgery residency at the University of Iowa Hospitals and Clinics, as well as a transplant research fellowship at the Starzl Transplant Institute at the University of Pittsburgh. He then completed a two-year transplantation surgery fellowship at the Massachusetts General Hospital, Harvard Medical School, and then joined the Division of Solid Organ Transplantation and Hepatobiliary Surgery at the University of Rochester Medical Center as an associate professor of surgery. He has currently moved back to Greece, where he is a professor of transplantation surgery and chief at the Department of Transplantation Surgery at the Aristotle University of Thessaloniki School of Medicine and the Center for Research and Innovation in Solid Organ Transplantation. He has published over 200 papers in peer-reviewed journals and PubMed, as well as 35 book chapters with an H-index of 29. He has edited six books and is a reviewer for 30 international journals and is on the editorial board of several others, including *International Surgery* and *Annals of Surgical Oncology*. The recipient of awards such as the Edward E. Mason Award for excellence in patient care and education, he is a member of several professional organizations including the TTS, the American Society of Transplant Surgeons, the Association for Academic Surgery, the International College of Surgeons, American College of Surgeons, International Liver Transplantation Society, Society for Laparoscopic Surgeons, and International HepaticoPancreaticoBiliary Association. He is also the recipient of the American College of Surgeons International Guest Scholarship. He has served as a member of multiple committees, including the International Relations Committee of the American College of Surgeons and the International Relations Committee of the American HepaticoPancreaticoBiliary Association (AHPBA). Currently the president of the Greek Chapter of the International College of Surgeons, he has served as World President of the International College of Surgeons and Chair of the International Relations Committee of the American College of Surgeons. He has served as a member of the AHPBA and the IHPBA Education and Training Committees the E-AHPBA Education Committee (Training Program Accreditation), the ASTS CME Committee, and the AASLD Training and Workforce Committee. He is also a member of the executive council of the Hellenic Surgical Society and president of the Hellenic Transplantation Society. Clinical and research interests include hepatobiliary surgery, primary and secondary hepatic malignancies, ischemia/reperfusion injury, and solid organ transplantation, as well as medical and surgical education and the use of technology, including applications of artificial technology and 3D printing in surgery.

Contents

Preface

Liver transplantation has always been one of the most interesting and challenging fields of medicine and surgery. It is a field that has made tremendous strides during the last few decades through the combined input and efforts of scientists from various specialties including surgeons, hepatologists, nephrologists, immunologists, ethicists, and infectious disease specialists. What started as a dream of pioneers has become a reality for the thousands of our patients whose lives can now be saved and improved. However, at the same time the challenges remain significant, and so do the expectations, for what was once an experimental treatment could eventually become the future of medicine, if you add to this scientifically explosive mix the rapid technological progress that we are witnessing with artificial intelligence, 3D printing, and extended reality.

In this book, with the contribution of an excellent group of world authorities in the field of liver transplantation, the different types of organ donors are presented along with the effect that machine perfusion will have on their utilization. Additionally, the future of liver transplantation is discussed, including the use of molecular technologies for diagnosis and organ function prediction and the most current criteria for liver transplantation in the case of hepatocellular carcinoma.

Overall, this book represents a true tour-de-force of a variety of topics in liver transplantation. It should be stressed that the intended audience is scientists, physicians, and surgeons of different specialties which all have in common an interest in transplantation and improving the lives of our patients.

Georgios Tsoulfas, MD, Ph.D., FICS, FACS
Professor of Transplantation Surgery,
Chief Department of Transplantation Surgery,
Center for Research and Innovation in Solid Organ Transplantation,
Aristotle University of Thessaloniki School of Medicine,
Thessaloniki, Greece

Section 1

Introduction – Overview of Liver Transplantation

Chapter 1

Introductory Chapter: Liver Transplantation – The Path to a Bright Future!

Georgios Tsoulfas

1. Introduction

1.1 Evolution of liver transplantation

Liver transplantation by all accounts represents the pinnacle of surgical procedures. The reason is that the concept of saving a human life by removing a diseased organ and replacing it with one from another human excites the human imagination, in addition to the fact that the recipient is usually a patient with cirrhosis and portal hypertension, which makes any type of intervention critical. When the first liver transplantation was performed on March 1st 1963 in Colorado, USA, by Thomas E. Starzl, it was a groundbreaking event that shook the world [1]. However, none of the first five patients undergoing a liver transplantation at that time survived longer than 23 days. This brought severe criticism, and if it wasn't for the tenacious spirit and stubbornness of Dr. Starzl, we would probably not be where we are today. The challenges were numerous during the first decade and included technical considerations, immunosuppression medication to overcome rejection, and the definition of brain death and ability to identify suitable donors and recipients, among others. The latter meant that it was critical to understand what was the best timing for a liver transplant, meaning that if it occurred too early, then it would not signify the best use of the liver graft, and if it occurred too late in the disease progression, then it would not benefit the recipient.

Over time, liver transplantation overcame the initial appearance of an experimental procedure and became the mainstay treatment for a variety of diseases and tumors of the liver. What this meant was that, eventually, it became a victim of its own success, as the increased acceptance by the medical and surgical world led to increased indications and need, which made the donor identification and management the limiting factor. So, the next hurdle to overcome was finding ways to increase the number of hepatic grafts, as well as improve the allocation process. The lack of donors led to the use of hepatic grafts from donors after circulatory death (DCD), from extended criteria (the definition of which is still a matter of significant debate) donors, and the practice of splitting a hepatic graft into two, so that the smaller one could be used for a child and the larger one for an adult recipient. Additionally, there have been, and continue to be, efforts to develop xenotransplantation, with the hope that it would provide an endless supply of donors, although the obstacles there (at least till recently) have been very high, given the immunological and biological differences across different species. These challenges and the difficulty of finding a proper graft for a child in need played a major role in the development of living donor liver transplantation, which represents a big step if we consider that the living donor undergoes a high-risk surgical procedure without any benefit to their health. Living donor liver transplantation evolved at different speeds in various parts of the world, with cultural and religious beliefs playing a significant role. Apart from the issue of finding a donor, given the scarcity of hepatic grafts, the question of proper allocation was just as important. This was addressed over time with an effort to identify an objective manner to prioritize the need and place on the waiting list, as in liver transplantation, the important issue is not how long someone is on the waiting list, but rather how advanced the liver disease is. The advent of the Model for End-stage Liver Disease (MELD) changed the landscape and over time continues to evolve as a very useful tool in prioritizing patients on the list [2].

The continued progress in the development of liver transplantation has led us to today where we are witnessing a further rapid expansion of liver transplantation globally, with certain key aspects, which can lead to a very promising future. Specifically:

a. Increasing number and quality of donors: an important development toward increasing both the number and quality of available hepatic grafts has been the increasing use of machine perfusion in liver transplantation, which is taking over liver transplantation in the last decade. The goal is to improve organ storage as well as organ quality, especially in recipients with extended criteria or suboptimal livers [3]. This is a work in progress as different types of machine perfusion are being used and evaluated, such as normothermic machine perfusion (NMP), hypothermic oxygenated machine perfusion (HOPE), and normothermic regional perfusion (NRP) compared to the more "traditional" static cold storage [4–6]. Although, the use of machine perfusion has decreased the number of discarded livers, especially in cases such as DCD donors, there still remain a lot of questions in terms of identifying the advantages and disadvantages of the different modalities, or even combinations thereof [7].

b. Xenotransplantation: with the help of genetic scientists, it has been possible to overcome significant immunologic hurdles in xenotransplantation, as shown by the recent groundbreaking efforts, which have renewed the faith in this overall approach [8].

c. The role of technology: technology moves at a lightning speed in our days, as evidenced by the leaps and bounds of artificial intelligence (AI), the increasing use of 3D printing in medicine and surgery, and the introduction of augmented and virtual reality from the lab to the bedside [9]. The technological imperative makes it crucial that future physicians in transplantation not only acknowledge its existence but also actively make an effort to understand it and make the best use of this huge potential.

The developments mentioned above are critical to the future of liver transplantation; however, what has led to them and what will continue to be the driving force in the future is the realization that liver transplantation is truly a multidisciplinary field, where surgery, hepatology, anesthesiology, intensive care, engineering, informatics, ethics, and law are only some of the fields that have collaborated to get us where we are. Acknowledging, appreciating, and further pursuing this collaboration is the path to a bright future!

Author details

Georgios Tsoulfas
Chief Department of Transplantation Surgery, Center for Research and Innovation in Solid Organ Transplantation, Aristotle University School of Medicine, Thessaloniki, Greece

*Address all correspondence to: tsoulfasg@auth.gr

References

[1] Meirelles RF Jr, Salvalaggio P, de Rezende MB, et al. Liver transplantation: History, outcomes and perspectives. Einstein (Sao Paulo). 2015;**13**(1):149-152

[2] Trivedi HD. The evolution of the MELD score and its implications in liver transplant allocation: A beginner's guide for trainees. American College of Gastroenterology Case Reports Journal. 2022;**9**(5):e00763. E collection

[3] Tingle SJ, Dobbins JJ, Thompson ER, et al. Machine perfusion in liver transplantation. Cochrane Database of Systematic Reviews. 2023;**9**(9):CD014685

[4] Feng GY, Feng X, Tao J, et al. Benefits of hypothermic oxygenated perfusion versus static cold storage in liver transplant: A comprehensive systematic review and meta-analysis. Journal of Clinical and Experimental Hepatology. 2024;**14**(3):101337

[5] Rawashdeh B, Kim J, Prasad R, Cooper M. A global overview on the evolution, debate and research output on liver transplant perfusion machines. Experimental and Clinical Transplantation. 2024;**22**(1):35-42

[6] Muller X, Rossignol G, Mohkam K, Mabrut JY. Back to basics: Liver graft ischemia in the era of machine perfusion. Transplantation. 2024. DOI: 10.1097/TP.0000000000004912 [Online ahead of print]

[7] Ghinolfi D, Patrono D, De Carlis R, et al. Liver transplantation with uncontrolled versus controlled DCD donors using normothermic regional perfusion and ex-situ machine perfusion. Liver Transplantation. 2024;**30**(1):46-60

[8] Anand RP, Layer JV, Heja D, et al. Desing and testing of a humanized porcine donor for xenotransplantation. Nature. 2023;**622**:393-401

[9] Christou CD, Tsoulfas G. Role of three-dimensional printing and artificial intelligence in the management of hepatocellular carcinoma: Challenges and opportunities. World Journal of Gastrointestinal Oncology. 2022;**14**(4):765-793

Section 2

Donation Issues in Liver Transplantation

Chapter 2

Deceased by Brain Death Liver Transplant vs. Living Donor Transplant/Putting Deceased Donor on Pump

Ahmed H. Abdelwahed and Elizabeth Richardson

Abstract

A written discussion of deceased by brain death vs. living donor and the use of the pump in deceased donor in liver transplant. Overview of living donor evaluation and potential contraindications to living donor liver transplant. Include a brief discussion on expanded donors in deceased donor liver transplant including steatotic livers and livers from donors of advanced age. It could also include a discussion on deceased by cardiac death liver transplant donation and potential complications from utilizing expanded criteria donors. Comparison of outcomes, advantages, and disadvantages between deceased by brain decath (DBD) and living donor transplant. Describe how the use of a pump expands the use of available livers. Also, review mechanisms of available pump technologies.

Keywords: DBD, pump, living donor, liver transplant, deceased donor

1. Introduction

Liver transplantation is a life-saving procedure for patients with complications of end-stage liver disease and stage T2 hepatocellular carcinoma. In 2017, deaths due to cirrhosis constituted 2.4% of total deaths globally, a rise from 1.9% in 1990. Leading causes include hepatitis B, hepatitis C, alcohol-associated liver disease, and non-alcoholic fatty liver disease (NAFLD) [1]. On the other hand, hepatocellular carcinoma is the sixth-most frequent new tumor, with more than 800,000 new cases diagnosed yearly and over 900,000 deaths every year, making it the fourth most common cause of cancer death [2]. The burden of these diseases makes the supply of liver organs for transplant outstrip the demand. The greatest challenge lies in the fact that there are not enough livers for all the potential patients that could benefit from liver transplantation. Today, in the United States, there are around 10,500 patients on the waiting list for liver transplants. Yet only 7000 liver transplants were performed in 2023. In 2017, >14,000 patients were on a waiting list, and only 8000 transplants were performed [3].

The consequences of being on a waiting list are not entirely favorable, with a mortality rate of 20–25% of waitlisted patients. A lengthy period of waiting can lead to further disease progression and debilitation before a transplant can be performed. Furthermore, severe deterioration can lead to the inability to perform the transplant and reserve the organ for other patients who might get the best outcomes [4].

It is well-known that most organs for transplantation are procured from deceased by brain death (DBD) donors. However, several challenges have emerged as the demand for liver transplants continues to rise and outweighs the supply. Improvement in safety, fortunately, has decreased the number of severe head injuries in young fit adults who used to be suitable DBD donors [5]. Furthermore, there has been an increase in the donor pool from an aging population with multiple co-morbidities. These challenges led to a shift in the paradigm to increase the donor pool. In the United States, there has been an 18% increase in liver transplant rate in the past 5 years, with the bigger proportion of the increase occurring among living donors, higher-risk donors as donation after circulator death (DCD), and the use of marginal grafts that carry technical challenge given age or risk of transmission of infection or malignancy [6]. Distinct types of liver transplants, outcomes, challenges, and future prospects will be discussed in this chapter.

2. Organ procurement

With the increased demand for liver transplants, proper organ procurement from a deceased donor remains an especially crucial step for a successful liver transplantation. Brain death is associated with various hemodynamic changes including hormonal, metabolic, and inflammatory changes in body organs. These changes might lead to increased immunogenicity and a higher risk of graft rejection. Hence, the optimal management of the organs might ensure their optimal function after transplantation [7]. The surgical technique for liver procurement includes warm and cold dissections. Warm dissection has the advantage of perfusion after identifying the vascular structures. However, the cold dissection technique might provide the benefits of shorter operation time and less organ damage through rapid procurement [8]. The classical method of preservation is keeping the liver in a basin that is filled with histidine-tryptophan-ketoglutarate solution (HTK). The first bag is sealed and placed in a second bag filled with cold normal saline or slushed ice, then placed in a third bag. The three-layered bag is finally placed in a heat preservation container box filled with ice for transportation [7]. New advances in liver preservation and transportation will be discussed later in this book chapter.

3. Overview of organ utilization

3.1 The use of marginal grafts

In the United States, one in four patients on the waiting list die before undergoing a transplant (12%) or become too sick to undergo liver transplantation (LT) (13%) [3]. This sad consequence of the disparity between the demand and supply of liver donation has emerged new prospects in expanding the donor pool and minimizing the rate of discarded organs. Central to these efforts is the liberalization of the acceptance criteria and use of the so-called "Marginal Livers" (MLs). Historically, that included livers that confer increased risk for poor graft and patient survival for various reasons including older age of donors (more than 70 years), DCD grafts, Viremic patients, livers split between two recipients, steatotic livers and the so-called "livers that nobody wants" which are livers that were initially declined by many centers before finally getting accepted by another center [9]. Listed Liver transplant patients who refused marginal organs have increased mortality risk compared to patients who accepted one [10].

3.2 Older age donors

Earlier data that looked at the utility of using marginal donors for liver transplantation associated older age (more than 70 years old) with worse outcomes and less chance for graft survival [11]. The explanation was that older livers have higher rates of steatosis, which might potentiate cold preservation injury. Some other data showed decreased adenosine triphosphate (ATP) capacity after reperfusion, which is thought to decrease the regenerative capacity [12]. This early data increased the aversion to elderly donors' livers, and they are usually discarded [13].

A retrospective study by Halazun et al. [13] looked at the utilization of using older donors by looking at the outcomes of 3104 patients who received livers from donors more than the age of 70 years old. The authors demonstrated that although unadjusted outcomes of elderly grafts are inferior to those of younger donors, recipient factors like hepatitis c and prior surgery played a bigger role in impacting survival more than donors themselves. They further showed that cold ischemic time (CIT) is the only donor factor that impacted the outcome. Worse outcomes are associated with CIT time of more than 8 hours. The authors hypothesized that livers of older donors are underutilized.

Another systemic review looked at the outcomes in patients who received livers from octogenarian patients and showed non-inferior short and medium-term graft survival. However, they reported increased biliary complications [14]. Another cohort study looked at the trend of transplantation of liver grafts from older donors from 2003 to 2016. In 3350 liver-only recipients, the authors demonstrated that despite improvement in graft survival and decreased mortality, the rate of discarded organs increased [15]. These studies showed that it is reasonable to expand the donor pool by using grafts from older people [13–15].

3.3 Hepatitis C liver grafts

Historically, hepatitis C virus (HCV) viremic grafts used to decline and be discarded [16]. The development of Direct antiviral agents (DAAs) has revolutionized the treatment of HCV and consequently increased the potential of using HCV viremic grafts. A landmark clinical trial by Wooley et al. looked at the outcome of 44 adults without HCV who received heart or lung transplantation from HCV-positive patients. They initiated sofosbuvir-velpatasvir, A DAA regimen, preemptively a few hours after the transplantation and for 4 weeks. After 6 months, the authors demonstrated that 100% of the first 35 patients who received transplantation were alive with excellent graft survival and had undetectable HCV viral load [17]. A limitation of this study was the small number of patients enrolled. The American Association for the Study of Liver Diseases (AASLD) endorsed HCV viremic donors as an option for use by HCV-negative recipients [18]. A study by Cotter et al. in 2021 showed a 35-fold increase in HCV positive over 4 years, from 8 in 2016 to 280 in 2019. The author demonstrated excellent graft survival in one and 2 years. Furthermore, when adjusted for other recipients' and donors' attributes, HCV viremic grafts were not predictive of patient or graft survival [19].

3.4 DCD patients

Historically, organs were obtained from patients after cardiac arrest. In 1968, the committee of Harvard Medical School promoted the acceptance of brain death [20]. With that recognition, DBD gained widespread acceptance and constituted the majority of transplants. As the available pool of liver remains insufficient to meet the demands, DCD LT has grown to be an effective and acceptable mechanism to expand the donor pool and decrease waitlist mortality [21]. The utilization of DCD livers has increased more than sixfold, from 1.9% in 2002 to 12.1% in 2016 [22]. DCD LT differs from DBD donations based on the warm ischemic time (WIT), which is the time between cardiac death and organ cooling during procurement. The classification of DCD donors was originally described by the international workshop on non-heartbeating donors held in Maastricht in 1995. The classification included four categories, which are dead upon arrival, death after resuscitation, donors who are awaiting cardiac arrest, and cardiac arrest after brain death [23]. To further categorize donors who are expected to be exposed to a longer duration of ischemic time, the definitions of controlled and uncontrolled were added. The controlled definition included the first two categories [24]. A 2017 propensity-match study that compared the outcomes of liver transplantation between 300 DBD and DCD showed 5-year graft survival of 73.9% in DBD group versus 70.1% in the DCD group [25]. Another study by Abt et al. demonstrated that DBD liver transplant patients had better 1- and 3-year graft survival of 80.4 and 72.1% versus 70.2 and 63.3% in DCD LT patients [26].

Risk factors for donors that may lead to complications include donor age of over 50, weight over 100 kilograms, and warm ischemic time of over 30 minutes [27]. A retrospective review by Foley et al. looked at long-term outcomes of 85 patients who had DCD liver transplants and showed that CIT for more than 8 hours is a strong predictor for the development of ischemic cholangiopathy [28]. Recipients' risk factors that might be more associated with complications include BMI of more than >30, hepatitis C positive recipients, and high model end-stage liver disease. Various complications have been associated with DCD LT, such as primary non-function, delayed graft rejection, and hepatic artery thrombosis [29]. A study by Croom et al. revealed that 25% of DCD liver transplants had biliary complications compared with 13% in the DBD group. A possible biliary complication is ischemic cholangiopathy [30]. Proposed methods to improve outcomes in DCD LT like machine perfusion will be discussed in detail later in this chapter.

3.5 Steatotic liver grafts

Given the pandemic of obesity and the increased prevalence of metabolic-associated dysfunction steatohepatitis (MASH), donor liver steatosis is becoming an increasingly common challenge that is facing the transplant community. The presence of moderate (more than 30% of Macro steatosis) has been associated with increased graft failure and primary non-function. However, the data has not been consistent [31]. Several studies showed that severe steatosis >60% has a higher risk of complications. A study by McCormack et al. demonstrated a higher rate of renal failure, long-term intensive care unit (ICU) stay (more than 21 days), and prolonged hospital stay (more than 40 days) in patients who received severely steatotic livers compared to the control group without severe steatosis. However, the sixty-day mortality and the 3-year patient survival rates were comparable [32]. Another study compared the outcomes between liver grafts with moderate steatosis and without steatosis after cardiac death showed that 90-day, 1-year, and 3-year survival rates in patients were similar (75 vs. 85.9%, 75 vs. 78.1%, 68.8 vs. 71.9%). The 90-day and 3-year graft survival were 75 vs. 84.4% and 68.8 vs. 68.8% between the two groups [33].

A meta-analysis in 2019 that looked at the impact of mild, moderate, and severe steatosis on liver transplantation showed there was no difference between mild and no steatosis groups in primary non-function (PNF) and early graft dysfunction. The PNF rate was significantly higher in moderately and severe steatosis than in the no steatosis group. However, graft survival and patient survival were similar in both groups. The authors concluded that liver with mild steatosis were safe liver grafts. Moderate and severe liver steatosis, although controversial, could produce a favorable outcome with strict protocols to keep CIT as short as possible, which might potentially expand donors' pool of livers and provide a potential solution for this shortage [34].

3.6 Split liver transplantation

In Split liver transplantation (SLT), Donor livers are classically split into a smaller left lateral segment which is typically used for children LT, and a larger right tri-segment for adults. This led to a reduction in the pediatric waiting list mortality [35]. Further advancement enabled the use of two hemi-liver grafts, a left lobe (segment I-IV) and a right lobe (segment V-VIII), for transplant in two adult-sized recipients. This technique is underutilized, given technical challenges and the risk of reducing an excellent graft into two marginal grafts [36]. Initial experiences of split liver grafting showed increased morbidity and mortality in adult recipients [37]. A multicenter retrospective study compared the overall graft survival in situ split liver extended right grafts (SL-ERGs) between 1997 and 2004 and thereafter. The 1,3,5 overall graft survival was significantly higher in more recent transplantation. In multivariate analysis, the main prognostic factor of graft survival was a total ischemic time of less than 8 hours. The donor age of more than 60 years was associated with increased graft failure. The study suggested that SL-ERGs might not be considered as marginal grafts in experienced LT centers if appropriate precautions are taken in choosing appropriate donors [38].

More research is needed to investigate the outcomes of hemi-liver split liver transplantation. A multicenter study by Aseni et al. compared patient and graft survival outcomes between recipients who had an adult-to-adult split liver transplant (AASLT) compared with recipients of a whole graft. The study revealed a higher complication rate and inferior 5-year survival rate in SLT when compared with whole liver transplantation [39]. A recent study compared adult liver hemi transplantation (AHLT) versus adult with whole liver transplantation (AWHLT) in both patients with MELD scores of more and less than 30.

Among patients with model of end-stage liver disease (MELD) >30 and < 30, AHLT correlated with higher WIT, operative and hospitalization time, and intra-operative blood loss. In MELD score > 30, the 5-year survival year in the AWHLT group was significantly higher. However, there was no significant difference between survival outcomes in patients with MELD scores less than 30 [40].

Criteria for Split liver transplantation are strict, and only hemodynamically stable cadaveric donors are eligible for split liver transplantation. Criteria for left lateral splitting include age less than 55 years; fatty degeneration >30%; intensive care stay of less than 5 days; sodium level less than 160; serum glutamic pyruvic transaminase <60 U/L; gamma-glutamyl transpeptidase <50 U/L. The requirements are more strict when left/right full split is pursued with better outcomes when the donor age is less than 40, fatty degeneration is less than 10%, and ICU stay is less than 3 days [41].

A recent analysis of 37,333 liver transplants performed between 2010 and 2015 in the United States revealed that 2352 (6.3%) met the strict criteria of split liver transplant utilization. However, only 1418 livers (3.8%) were utilized for split liver transplantation. Two hundred ninety-nine children died on the waitlist who could have potentially benefited from split liver transplantation. The study suggested that split liver transplantation is an underutilized tool and should be promoted to decrease children's waitlist mortality [42].

4. Organ preservation in liver transplantation

4.1 Novel techniques in organ preservation methods

The research in the field of Dynamic organ preservation goes back to the last century. Thomas E. Starlz, a pioneer of liver transplantation, performed an ex vivo liver perfusion of a chimpanzee in an attempt for liver transplantation without a favorable outcome [43]. Despite being a hot topic at that time, the revolutionary development of the University of Wisconsin solution provided a safe, effective, and simple method of liver preservation, leaving machine perfusion aside, given its higher costs and complexity. Since then, static cold storage has become the gold standard method of liver and other organ preservation [44]. With the expansion of the use of marginal grafts to bridge the gap between the demand and available organs for liver transplantation, the need for reliable measures to assess liver quality prior to transplant has emerged. This has led to the development of new strategies of dynamic preservation, mainly aiming to improve organ viability, extend preservation time, and assess organ quality. The efforts in the development of machine liver perfusion were resuscitated [45].

There are two important distinguishing factors in liver machine perfusion, one is the temperature, and the second is the approach. The perfusate's temperature has a detrimental effect on the rate of metabolic functions in the liver, which is crucial for the intended metabolic effect. The first hypothermic liver machine perfusion device was introduced in humans in 2004 [46]. Liver perfusion in hypothermic conditions (below 12-degree Celsius) leads to a significant suppression of metabolic demands. The need for oxygenators versus perfusate oxygen was studied extensively, with the data revealing the clear metabolic need for oxygen during hypothermic conditions but at a low level. The perfusion during hypothermic machine, perfusion can be done via portal vein or dual perfusion through the portal vein and hepatic artery. In 2016, a study by Schlegel et al. revealed that a portal vein-only approach might be sufficient for hypothermic machine perfusion in DCD liver grafts [47].

In contrast, normothermic liver perfusion requires a very high metabolic demand with full availability of physiologic oxygen requirements and nutrients to keep the liver viable. In terms of achieving this level of perfusion, the machines are more complex and require dual perfusion lines for the portal vein and hepatic artery with readily available sensors for the metabolic demands and oxygen levels. Normothermic or sub-normothermic perfusions require red blood cells or artificial oxygen carriers, in contrast to the hypothermic oxygenated perfusion (HOPE) performed with high perfusate oxygen concentration. The first human application for normothermic machine liver perfusion was introduced in 2012 [48].

There are two main ex-situ perfusion approaches for livers that are essentially different in terms of timing and protective mechanism. The first method is the upfront machine perfusion immediately after procurement to replace classical cold static preservation. The organ in this approach is placed in a transportable device and undergoes continuous perfusion until the organ arrives at the recipient center and implantation occurs. This method requires complex and expensive systems to be used with blood products as the perfusate and typically includes normothermic or sub-normothermic perfusion [49]. A modification of this method is the normothermic regional perfusion (NRP), where perfusion is started earlier after the patient's cardiac arrest and cannulation. The perfusion is done in situ with the donor's blood for 2-4 hours before a decision is made regarding the procurement of the liver according to the liver enzymes and lactic acid values. This process aims to minimize the cold ischemic time [50].

The other liver machine perfusion approach is different in timing. It is usually applied after organ transportation at the recipient center. In this end-ischemic approach, the organs are usually perfused for a short time before transplantation using hypothermic, normothermic, or a combination of both in a process named controlled oxygenated rewarming. These techniques are less complex and less logistically challenging than upfront machine perfusion because there is no transportation of the machine perfusion device. However, it exposes the organ to a longer cold ischemic time, and subsequently, there is a risk for severe metabolic derangements, especially in higher-risk grafts [51].

4.2 Outcomes of transplantation after machine perfusion

As mentioned above, LT after DCD carries the risk of biliary complications including non-anastomotic biliary constrictions with studies showing cold ischemic time as an important factor in developing such complications [28, 29]. Machine perfusion transplantation aimed to decrease cold ischemic time and then decrease complications. Pre-clinical studies have shown that 2 hours of hypothermic machine perfusion (HMP) can restore mitochondrial functions and decrease the production of radical oxygen species that might damage the cells before transplantation [52].

The first clinical series done in human liver transplantation after hypothermic machine perfusion was done in 2010 by Guarrera et al. Transplant outcomes of 20 adult patients who received HMP-preserved livers were compared to a matching group of patients who received transplantation of livers after conventional cold storage. Early allograft dysfunction was seen in 5% of the HMP group and 25% in the control group, but the results were not statistically significant. Serum injury markers and hospital stay duration were significantly lower in the HMP group. This small, controlled pilot study demonstrated safety and feasibility and subsequently warranted further multicenter trials [53].

In 2017, Van Riijn and his colleagues completed a non-randomized controlled trial where they matched ten patients who received end-ischemic DHOPE-DCD (dual portal vein and hepatic artery hypothermic oxygenated machine perfusion of DCD liver grafts) to 20 patients who underwent static cold storage in the same center. Patients were matched for age, MELD score, and warm ischemic time and were followed for a year. The DHOPE recipients had statistically significantly lower alanine transferase (ALT) and gamma-glutamyl transferase (GGT). The one-year survival rate for patients and grafts was 100% in the DHOPE recipients. Five patients in the static cold storage group required retransplantation for non-anastomotic biliary stricture, while none of the DHOPE treated livers required retransplantation. However, this result was not statistically significant. The authors noted a significantly higher incidence of hypokalemia in the DHOPE group. This study was challenged by the very small number of patients and the use of historical controls [54].

In 2019, Schlegel et al. looked at the long-term outcomes (5 years) of DCD liver transplants after donor organs had been treated with hypothermic oxygenated perfusion. The study compared 50 hope-treated DCD patients from Zurich to 50 DBD patients and 50 untreated DCD patients from the United Kingdom. The patients were matched for recipient age, cold ischemic time, and low MELD scores. The overall donor-recipient risk based on the UK DCD risk score was higher in the hope-treated patients given older donor ages and longer warm ischemic time. Despite the higher risk, hope-treated DCD patients achieved a similar graft survival outcome to the standard DBD transplants. The number of non-anastomotic strictures (NAS) was more than double in the untreated DCD group compared with the hope-treated group. Graft loss due to non-tumor causes occurred in 4 out of 50 patients in the hope-treated group compared to 16 patients in the untreated group. (8 vs. 32% with a P-value of 0.005). On a sub-group analysis censored for tumor death, the five-year graft survival was 94% in hope-treated grafts vs. 78% in untreated grafts (P = 0.024).

The study had some limitations; 70% of the recipients in the hope-treated group had hepatocellular carcinoma, and the exclusion of tumor-related graft failure could have potentially skewed the results. The perioperative protocols were different in both centers between Zurich and Birmingham. In addition, the immunosuppressive regimen was also different. These differences need to be considered and can present a limitation for the clinical significance of this trial [55].

In 2021, Czigany et al. conducted a prospective, multicentric, randomized controlled trial where 46 patients DCD LT patients were assigned to HOPE vs. static cold storage (SCS). Peak ALT value after 7 days was the primary endpoint. The authors demonstrated a 47% decrease in peak serum ALT level in the Hope group. They also showed a significant reduction in the 90-day complications, with 44% in the Hope group vs. 74% in the SCS group, in addition to a shorter ICU stay. A trend of reduced early allograft dysfunction was observed in the HOPE group but was not statistically significant. The perioperative and immunosuppression protocols were similar and standardized between the two groups of this study; however, the participating centers used different surgical techniques per their local protocols [56].

In a multicenter-controlled trial, Van Riijn et al. randomly assigned patients who were undergoing transplantation from DCD patients to receive livers after DHOPE treatment vs. SCS. The study included 160 patients, of whom 78 patients were assigned machine-perfused livers, and 78 were assigned SCS livers. The study was conducted in six liver transplantation centers in Europe. The primary endpoint of the study was the incidence of symptomatic non-anastomotic biliary strictures after 6 months of the transplantation. The criteria for NAS were specified as narrowing or irregularity of the intrahepatic or extrahepatic donor bile ducts, seen using cholangiography in the combination of clinical symptoms or a cholestatic pattern of the liver enzymes. The images were interpreted by two different radiologists who were blinded to the allocation of the patients. NAS biliary stricture occurred in 6% of the DHOPE-treated group vs. 18% in the untreated arm (P = 0.03). The authors also demonstrated a reduction of 15% in the incidence of the post perfusion syndrome between the two groups, with 12% in the DHOPE group and 27% in the control group. In addition, early allograft dysfunction (EAD) occurred in 26% of the machine-perfused livers vs.

40% in the untreated livers. In this trial, the machine perfusion had no effect on the ICU duration stay, patients, or graft survival [57].

Normothermic ex-situ perfusion might give a chance to assess the viability of the liver before transplantation. In 2018, Watson et al. studied the characteristics of 47 liver perfusion, of which 22 resulted in liver transplantation. The authors demonstrated that liver viability during NMP can be assessed through a combination of lactate clearance, glucose release, maintenance of acid-base balance, and transaminase release. They also showed that PH can be a valuable prognostication for bile integrity. Bile PH measured in 16 out of 22 transplanted livers identified three livers that developed cholangiopathy, which was less than 7.4. Biliary PH was measured in 11 research livers; four achieved a PH of more than 7.5 and had minimal stromal necrosis of the intrahepatic ducts on histological examination [58].

The first randomized trial was completed in 2018 by Nasralla et al. In this trial, the authors compared normothermic machine liver preservation with the conventional cold static methods. Livers from DCD and DBD were included, and 334 livers were randomized between the two arms of the study. The primary endpoint of this study was the difference in serum aspartate transaminase (AST) within 7 days of the transplant between the two groups. Secondary endpoints included early allograft dysfunction (EAD), biliary strictures seen on MRCP after 6 months of transplant, hospital stay, graft survival and patient survival. The Peak AST after 7 days of transplant was reduced by 49.4% in the NMP group, disclosing a difference of 477 IU/L between the two groups. The rate of EAD was also significantly lower in the NMP. The study, however, failed to show a significant difference in biliary complications and patient or graft survival despite including mainly low-risk livers and choosing recipients of lower MELD scores. Another weakness is choosing AST as a primary outcome, which is a weak parameter of liver injury after transplantation [49].

In 2022, Quintini et al. demonstrated the role of enhancing graft preservation, extending viability by evaluating previously discarded livers. Twenty-one human livers declined for transplantation were enrolled to be assessed for normothermic machine perfusion. Livers were subjected to the proprietary device without issues. Six livers were ultimately excluded from NMP after failing to meet the criteria for transplantation with failure to clear lactate, limited bile production, or moderate macrosteatosis. Fifteen livers were transplanted successfully. No intraoperative or early major postoperative complication occurred in any of the recipients. No primary non-function occurred in any of the patients. Seven patients developed early allograft dysfunction but had fast recovery. Only one patient developed cholangiopathy in 4 months, and the rest of the patients had good liver functions with a follow-up time of 2 months to 14 months. The authors demonstrated that the viability criteria can be expanded. However, the study was done in one single center, and the small sample is a limitation for the reliability of the study [59].

Recently, Markmann et al. conducted a multicenter randomized controlled trial across 20 liver transplant programs in the United States. The trial compared the outcomes of 300 recipients of livers preserved using either normothermic machine perfusion or ischemic cold storage. The authors demonstrated a significant reduction in early organ dysfunction in the NMP group (18 vs. 31%). The NMP-preserved livers showed a significantly decreased incidence of ischemic reperfusion injury (6 vs. 13%). In addition, ischemic biliary complications were lower after 6 and 12 months in the NMP group. The 1-year graft survival rate was comparable between the two groups after 1 year [60].

5. Living donor liver transplantation

Despite the advancement in the field of liver transplantation, organ shortage remains an important challenge. Approaches to overcoming this issue include the use of marginal organs as organs from DCD patients, the use of machine perfusion in suboptimal grafts, and organs from patients who are infected with hepatitis C or HIV, which has been explained earlier in this chapter. With growing experience, living donor liver transplantation has become an established viable strategy to mitigate organ shortage.

Living donor liver transplantation (LDLT) may offer a chance of survival for patients with end-stage liver disease and hepatocellular carcinoma who are at a high risk of death while waiting for a suitable liver on the waiting list. Recent studies showed that LDLT could offer multiple theoretical advantages over DBD LT including shorter wait time and possible better graft quality [4]. A comparison of outcomes with DBT LT will take place by the end of this chapter.

The idea of LDLT was proposed as early as 1969 by Smith B., with the first attempt carried out by Raia et al. in 1989. The first successful LDLT was reported by Strong et al. in 1989 when they transplanted a liver from a living donor to her son in Australia [61]. Although the LT technique started earlier in the West, it quickly became the most common form of liver transplantation in Asia, with over 90% of the transplants performed using grafts that are commonly donated by relatives and friends. LDLT developed as a standard of treatment out of necessity due to the very limited number of deceased brain liver donors. The unique cultures, demographics, politics, and religion made the acceptance of DDLT remain limited despite its legalization in different countries [62].

LDLT has been considered a feasible and effective technique for decades, but it needs significant resource utilization and surgical expertise. In addition, donor safety, small size, and biliary complications remain major obstacles [63].

5.1 Donor safety in living donor transplant

Yee Lee et al. conducted a worldwide survey of the programs that perform LDLT to determine the incidence of mortality, morbidity, and near-miss events. The response rate was 48% (71 programs) that performed donor hepatectomy 11,533 times. They were able to give information regarding the case volume, demographics, graft types, morbidity mortality, and near-miss events. The study was able to generate reliable data demonstrating a morbidity rate of 24%, with 0.04% of patients requiring liver transplantation. The donor mortality was 0.2%, with most deaths occurring in the first 60 days after the procedure [64]. The adult-to-adult living donor liver transplantation cohort study (A2ALL) analyzed 760 donors. The no-go rate of donation was 2.6%, which was primarily due to findings in the operating room. The authors demonstrated a mortality rate of 0.4% and an overall complication rate of 40%. Serious complications that led to liver failure or death occurred in 1.1%. The most common complications included infections (12%), Biliary leak (9%), and incisional hernia in 6% of patients. The study suggested a trend of higher complication rates in left lobe donations, but the number of donors was very small (33 patients) which made the interpretation of the data challenging [65]. A study that looked at the quality of life for donors 11 years after donation using the health-related quality of life (HRQOL) surveys in living donors showed that they experience a higher quality of life compared to the general population [66]. Muzaale et al. followed up on 4111 livers in the United

States between March 1994 and April 2003 and determined mortality using the Social Security death master file. The death rate was 1.7 per 1000 donors. The mortality of donors did not differ from healthy-matched individuals over a mean of 7.6 years. The rate of catastrophic events was 2.9 per 1000 donors, and five donors suffered from acute liver failure, where one improved, one passed, and three required DDLT salvage [67].

To maintain the safety and well-being of donors, LDLT centers have established strict criteria for selecting suitable donors. The donor age, degree of steatosis, and remnant liver volume (RLV) are important influential factors. The RLV should be fully functioning without venous congestion. In most LDLT centers, 30% of the total liver volume is widely accepted as a safety margin for minimal RLV [68]. Steatosis can affect the donor's liver functions and ability to regenerate. Besides, it can affect the morbidity and mortality of recipients. There are no clear guidelines regarding the acceptable degree of steatosis for donation, but patients with more than 30% of steatosis are not accepted for right liver hepatectomy for safety concerns. However, the use of diet-treated donors might be feasible after their weight loss [69].

5.2 Statistics and indications

There have been more than 4600 adult LDLTs performed in the United States through 2015, constituting less than 5% of the total number of transplants performed annually. In 2013, 6455 liver transplantations were performed, all from deceased donors and only 252 (4%) from living donors. In the same year, among 166 liver transplant centers in the United States, only 43 centers performed living donor liver transplantation [70].

The organ allocation from deceased donors in the United States is based on the 11 regions of the United Network of Organ Sharing (UNOS), with the organ assignment mainly built around the MELD score except in some cases like fulminant liver hepatitis and liver primary non-function in the first week. The system allows for "the sickest first" policy where patients with the highest MELD score get priority. Exception points are given to conditions that may hasten mortality without a high MELD score, like hepatocellular carcinoma, cystic fibrosis, and hepato-pulmonary syndrome [71].

Given the current allocation system, LDLT Is generally indicated to patients with end-stage cirrhosis with complications like ascites without a high MELD score, hepatocellular carcinoma (HCC) patients who do not meet criteria for LDLT, or in regions where wait time would exceed 12 months; other indications include cirrhosis with a low MELD score but significantly decreased quality of life, cholestatic liver disease with a low MELD score and recurrent cholangitis [72].

5.3 Outcomes in living donor liver transplantation in comparison with DBD (Deceased by brain death) patients

The adult-to-adult living donor liver transplantation (A2ALL) study demonstrated survival benefits compared to staying on the wait list for DDLT. A2ALL is a consortium of nine liver transplant centers created to conduct retrospective and prospective studies that looked at the outcomes of both donors and recipients in the period between 1998 and 2008 [73]. A subsequent study in 2005 looked at the outcomes of 385 LDLT recipients and demonstrated ninety-day and 1-year graft survival rates of 87 and 81%, respectively. 13.2% of the grafts failed in the first 90 days. The most common complications included sepsis, primary non-function, and vascular thrombosis.

The authors demonstrated that age and cold ischemic time are important predictors of graft failure. Interestingly, the centers that had a higher volume of cases (more than 20 LDLT) had significantly lower risk of graft failure [74]. Another subsequent study by Berg et al., looked at 868 potential recipients of LDLT, of whom 712 underwent transplantation. Overall, recipients had 56% lower mortality when compared to patients on the waiting list for DDLT. In patients without HCC, there was a mortality benefit in both groups of MELD scores of more and less than 15. In patients with HCC, a benefit was seen for patients with a MELD score of more than 15 but was not seen in the group with a MELD score of less than 15 [75]. A study by Goldberg et al. demonstrated that LDLT might be superior to DDLT when performed in experienced centers. The 3-year graft survival was higher in the LDLT group vs. the DDLT group (78.9 vs. 77.7%) [76].

Regarding hepatitis C recipients, a study demonstrated no differences between LDLT and DDLT groups in graft survival when the living donor transplantation is done in experienced high-volume centers that had more than 20 LDLT [77].

A recent study by Cotter et al. compared the UNOS data of 2566 LDLT patients with propensity scores that matched DDLT patients from 2010 to 2019. The authors demonstrated a doubling of LDLT from around 200 to 440 in 2019. One-year and 5-year graft survival in LDLT recipients was 88.4 and 78.1% compared with 92.5 and 80.7% in matched DBD patients. Older age, recipient diabetes, and the requirement of life support were associated with higher mortality and worse graft functions. The centers with the highest volume of LDLT per unit time had significantly superior outcomes in one-year graft survival [78].

LDLT can offer a clinically safe addition to deceased liver transplantation and can help decrease the mortality of being on a waiting list. Future surgical innovations and efforts to increase the living donor's pool may foster the advancement of living donor liver transplantation in the United States in the future.

6. Conclusion

Liver transplantation has transformed the management of acute and chronic liver diseases. It is considered a life-saving procedure for patients with end-stage liver disease. Organ shortage remains a big challenge as the big burden of the disease makes the supply of liver organs for transplant outstrip the demand. Hence, to increase the donor pool, the use of marginal liver grafts has become an inevitable tool to overcome this shortage. These marginal grafts include grafts that historically conferred increased risk for poor graft and patient survival for various reasons including older age of donors (more than 70 years), DCD grafts, Viremic patients, livers split between two recipients, and steatotic livers. Several approaches have been developed to improve the outcomes of these marginal grafts. This progress is mainly aimed at decreasing cold and warm ischemic time. With the expansion in using marginal grafts, the need for reliable measures to assess liver grafts emerged. This has led to the development of new strategies of dynamic preservation, mainly aiming to improve organ viability, extend preservation time, and assess organ quality. Machine perfusion may allow for an increase in usable liver grafts and significantly improve outcomes. However, lack of financial support, knowledge, and difficulties in logistics are still important challenges for wider implementation. Living donor liver transplantation is another method to overcome the organ shortage that has been more developed recently with a subsequent increased rate of LDLT in the United States. LDLT may offer survival benefits for patients who are on the waiting list for liver transplantation. More research is required to further improve both donors' and recipients' safety and overcome technical challenges associated with LDLT. More studies to compare the outcomes of LDLT with DBD are needed to further delineate the risks and benefits for both donors and recipients.

Author details

Ahmed H. Abdelwahed[1*] and Elizabeth Richardson[2]

1 Department of Internal Medicine, University of Connecticut, USA

2 Hartford Hospital, Department of Gastroenterology, and Hepatology, USA

*Address all correspondence to: richardson.em@gmail.com

References

[1] GBD 2017 Cirrhosis Collaborators. The global, regional, and national burden of cirrhosis by cause in 195 countries and territories, 1990-2017: A systematic analysis for the global burden of disease study 2017. The Lancet. Gastroenterology & Hepatology. 2020;**5**(3):245-266. DOI: 10.1016/S2468-1253(19)30349-8. EPub 2020 Jan 22

[2] World Health Organization. Global cancer observatory. Available from: https://gco.iarc.fr/2022[Accessed: December 20, 2022]

[3] Available from: https://optn.transplant.hrsa.gov/data/view-data-reports/national-data/

[4] Humar A, Ganesh S, Jorgensen D, Tevar A, Ganoza A, Molinari M, et al. Adult living donor versus deceased donor liver transplant (LDLT versus DDLT) at a single center: Time to change our paradigm for liver transplant. Annals of Surgery. 2019;**270**(3):444-451. DOI: 10.1097/SLA.0000000000003463

[5] Burke NT, Maurice JB, Nasralla D, Potts J, Westbrook R. Recent advances in liver transplantation. Frontline Gastroenterology. 2021;**13**(1):57-63. DOI: 10.1136/flgastro-2020-101425

[6] Taylor R, Allen E, Richards JA, Goh MA, Neuberger J, Collett D, et al. Liver advisory group to NHS blood and transplant. Survival advantage for patients accepting the offer of a circulatory death liver transplant. Journal of Hepatology. 2019;**70**(5):855-865. DOI: 10.1016/j.jhep.2018.12.033. Epub 2019 Jan 11

[7] Patel MS, Abt PL. Current practices in deceased organ donor management. Current Opinion in Organ Transplantation. 2019;**24**(3):343-350. DOI: 10.1097/MOT.0000000000000638

[8] Choi YR, Lee K. Liver procurement. Korean. Journal of Transplantation. 2015;**29**:109-117. DOI: 10.4285/jkstn.2015.29.3.109

[9] Feng S, Goodrich NP, Bragg-Gresham JL, Dykstra DM, Punch JD, DebRoy MA, et al. Characteristics associated with liver graft failure: The concept of a donor risk index. American Journal of Transplantation. 2006;**6**(4):783-790. DOI: 10.1111/j.1600-6143.2006.01242.x. [Erratum in: American Journal of Transplantation 2018 Dec;18(12):3085]

[10] Croome KP, Lee DD, Pungpapong S, Keaveny AP, Taner CB. What are the outcomes of declining a public health service increased risk liver donor for patients on the liver transplant waiting list? Liver Transplant. 2018;**24**(4):497-504

[11] Busquets J, Xiol X, Figueras J, Jaurrieta E, Torras J, Ramos E, et al. The impact of donor age on liver transplantation: Influence of donor age on early liver function and on subsequent patient and graft survival. Transplantation. 2001;**71**:1765-1771

[12] Busuttil RW, Tanaka K. The utility of marginal donors in liver transplantation. Liver Transplantation. 2003;**9**(7):651-663. DOI: 10.1053/jlts.2003.50105

[13] Halazun KJ, Rana AA, Fortune B, Quillin RC, Verna EC, Samstein B, et al. No country for old livers? Examining and optimizing the utilization of elderly liver grafts. American Journal of Transplantation. 2018;**18**(3):669-678

[14] Domagala P, Takagi K, Ijzermans JN, Polak WG. Grafts from selected deceased donors over 80 years old can safely expand the number of liver transplants: A systematic review and meta-analysis. Transplantation Reviews (Orlando, Fla.). 2019;**33**(4):209-218. DOI: 10.1016/j.trre.2019.06.004. Epub 2019 Jul 2

[15] Haugen CE, Holscher CM, Luo X, et al. Assessment of trends in transplantation of liver grafts from older donors and outcomes in recipients of liver grafts from older donors, 2003-2016. JAMA Surgery. 2019;**154**(5):441-449. DOI: 10.1001/jamasurg.2018.5568

[16] Kapila N,Menon KVN, Al-Khalloufi K, Vanatta JM, Murgas C, Reino D, et al. Hepatitis C virus NAT-positive solid organ allografts transplanted into hepatitis C virus-negative recipients: A real-world experience. Hepatology. 2020;**72**(1):32-41. DOI: 10.1002/hep.31011. Epub 2020 Apr 15

[17] Woolley AE, Singh SK, Goldberg HJ, Mallidi HR, Givertz MM, Mehra MR, et al. Heart and lung transplants from HCV-infected donors to uninfected recipients. The New England Journal of Medicine. 2019;**380**(17):1606-1617. DOI: 10.1056/NEJMoa1812406. Epub 2019 Apr 3

[18] Ghany MG, Morgan TR, Panel A-IHCG. Hepatitis C guidance 2019 update: American association for the study of liver diseases-infectious diseases society of America recommendations for testing, managing, and treating hepatitis C virus infection. Hepatology. 2020;**71**(2):686-721

[19] Cotter TG, Aronsohn A, Reddy KG, Charlton M. Liver transplantation of HCV-viremic donors into HCV-negative recipients in the United States: Increasing frequency with profound geographic variation. Transplantation. 2021;**105**(6):1285-1290. DOI: 10.1097/TP.0000000000003382

[20] A definition of irreversible coma. Report of the ad hoc Committee of the Harvard medical school to examine the definition of brain death. Journal of the American Medical Association. 1968;**205**(6):337-340

[21] Tector AJ, Mangus RS, Chestovich P, Vianna R, Fridell JA, Milgrom ML, et al. Use of extended criteria livers decreases wait time for liver transplantation without adversely impacting posttransplant survival. Annals of Surgery. 2006;**244**(3):439-450. DOI: 10.1097/01.sla.0000234896.18207.fa

[22] Saidi RF, Markmann JF, Jabbour N, et al. The faltering solid organ donor pool in the United States (2001-2010). World Journal of Surgery. 2012;**36**(12):2909-2913. DOI: 10.1007/s00268-012-1748-0

[23] Kootstra G, Daemen JH, Oomen AP. Categories of non-heart-beating donors. Transplantation Proceedings. 1995;**27**(5):2893-2894

[24] Rodríguez-Sanjuán JC, Ruiz N, Miñambres E, Toledo E, González-Noriega M, Fernández-Santiago R, et al. Liver transplant from controlled cardiac death donors using normothermic regional perfusion: Comparison with liver transplants from brain dead donors. Transplantation Proceedings. Jan-Feb 2019;**51**(1):12-19. DOI: 10.1016/j.transproceed.2018.04.067. Epub 2018 Jun 28. PMID: 30655135

[25] Croome KP, Lee DD, Perry DK, Burns JM, Nguyen JH, Keaveny AP, et al. Comparison of longterm outcomes and quality of life in recipients of donation after cardiac death liver grafts with a propensity-matched cohort. Liver Transplantation. 2017;**23**(3):342-351. DOI: 10.1002/lt.24713

[26] Abt PL, Desai NM, Crawford MD, et al. Survival following liver

transplantation from non-heartbeating donors. Annals of Surgery. 2004;**239**(1):87-92. DOI: 10.1097/01.sla.0000103063.82181.2c

[27] Selck FW, Grossman EB, Ratner LE, Renz JF. Utilization, outcomes, and retransplantation of liver allografts from donation after cardiac death: Implications for further expansion of the deceased-donor pool. Annals of Surgery. 2008;**248**(4):599-607. DOI: 10.1097/SLA.0b013e31818a080e

[28] Foley DP, Fernandez LA, Leverson G, Anderson M, Mezrich J, Sollinger HW, et al. Biliary complications after liver transplantation from donation after cardiac death donors: An analysis of risk factors and long-term outcomes from a single center. Annals of Surgery. 2011;**253**(4):817-825. DOI: 10.1097/SLA.0b013e3182104784

[29] Eren EA, Latchana N, Beal E, Hayes D Jr, Whitson B, Black SM. Donations after circulatory death in liver transplant. Experimental and Clinical Transplantation. 2016;**14**(5):463-470

[30] Croome KP, McAlister V, Adams P, Marotta P, Wall W, Hernandez-Alejandro R. Endoscopic management of biliary complications following liver transplantation after donation from cardiac death donors. Canadian Journal of Gastroenterology. 2012;**26**(9):607-610

[31] Jackson KR, Long J, Philosophe B, Garonzik-Wang J. Liver transplantation using Steatotic grafts. Clinical Liver Disease (Hoboken). 2019;**14**(5):191-195. DOI: 10.1002/cld.847

[32] McCormack L, Petrowsky H, Jochum W, Mullhaupt B, Weber M, Clavien PA. Use of severely steatotic grafts in liver transplantation: A matched case-control study. Annals of Surgery. 2007;**246**(6):940-946. discussion 946-8. DOI: 10.1097/SLA.0b013e31815c2a3f

[33] Duan X, Yan L, Shen Y, Zhang M, Bai X, Liang T. Outcomes of liver transplantation using moderately steatotic liver from donation after cardiac death (DCD). Annals of Translational Medicine. 2020;**8**(18):1188. DOI: 10.21037/atm-20-5888

[34] Zhang QY, Zhang QF, Zhang DZ. The impact of steatosis on the outcome of liver transplantation: A meta-analysis. BioMed Research International. 2019;**2019**:3962785. DOI: 10.1155/2019/3962785

[35] Busuttil RW, Goss JA. Split liver transplantation. Annals of Surgery. 1999;**229**:313-321

[36] Hashimoto K, Eghtesad B. Split liver transplantation. In: Doria C, editor. Contemporary Liver Transplantation. Switzerland: Springer; 2016

[37] Emond JC, Whitington PF, Thistlethwaite JR, Cherqui D, Alonso EA, Woodle IS, et al. Transplantation of two patients with one liver. Analysis of a preliminary experience with 'split-liver' grafting. Annals of Surgery. 1990;**212**:14-22

[38] Maggi U, De Feo TM, Andorno E, Cillo U, De Carlis L, Colledan M, et al. Liver transplantation and intestine North Italy transplant study group. Fifteen years and 382 extended right grafts from in situ split livers in a multicenter study: Are these still extended criteria liver grafts? Liver Transplantation. 2015;**21**(4):500-511. DOI: 10.1002/lt.24070

[39] Aseni P, De Feo TM, De Carlis L, Valente U, Colledan M, Cillo U, et al. A prospective policy development to increase split-liver transplantation for 2 adult recipients: Results of a 12-year

multicenter collaborative study. Annals of Surgery. 2014;**259**(1):157-165. DOI: 10.1097/SLA.0b013e31827da6c9

[40] Kong L, Lv T, Jiang L, Yang J, Yang J. Outcomes of hemi-versus whole liver transplantation in patients from mainland China with high model for end-stage liver disease scores: A matched analysis. BMC Surgery. 2020;**20**(1):290. DOI: 10.1186/s12893-020-00965-8

[41] Broering DC, Schulte am Esch J, Fischer L, Rogiers X. Split liver transplantation.HPB(Oxford).2004;**6**(2):76-82. DOI: 10.1080/13651820310020774

[42] Perito ER, Roll G, Dodge JL, Rhee S, Roberts JP. Split liver transplantation and pediatric waitlist mortality in the United States: Potential for improvement. Transplantation. 2019;**103**(3):552-557. DOI: 10.1097/TP.0000000000002249

[43] Starzl TE. Experience in hepatic transplantation. In: Orthotopic Heterotransplantation. Philadelphia: WB Saunders Co; 1969. pp. 408-421

[44] Belzer FO, Kalayoglu M, Dalessandro AM, Pirsch JD, Sollinger HW, Hoffmann R, et al. Organ preservation: Experience with University of Wisconsin solution and plans for the future. Clinical Transplantation. 1990;**4**(2):73-77

[45] Panconesi R, Carvalho MF, Muiesan P, Dutkowski P, Schlegel A. Liver perfusion strategies: what is best and do ischemia times still matter? Current Opinion in Organ Transplantation. 1 Aug 2022;**27**(4):285-299. DOI: 10.1097/MOT.0000000000000963. Epub 2022 Jan 31. PMID: 35438271

[46] Morito N, Obara H, Matsuno N, Enosawa S, Furukawa H. Oxygen consumption during hypothermic and subnormothermic machine perfusions of porcine liver grafts after cardiac death. Journal of Artificial Organs. 2018;**21**(4):450-457

[47] Schlegel A, Kron P, De Oliveira ML, Clavien PA, Dutkowski P. Is single portal vein approach sufficient for hypothermic machine perfusion of DCD liver grafts? Journal of Hepatology. 2016;**64**(1):239-241

[48] Kamo N, Ke B, Busuttil RW, Kupiec-Weglinski JW. PTEN mediated akt/β-catenin/foxo1 signaling regulates innate immune responses in mouse liver ischemia/reperfusion injury. Hepatology. 2013;**57**(1):289-298

[49] Nasralla D, Coussios CC, Mergental H, et al. A randomized trial of normothermic preservation in liver transplantation. Nature. 2018;**557**:50-56. DOI: 10.1038/s41586-018-0047-9. Epub 2018 Apr 18

[50] Hessheimer AJ, Coll E, Torres F, et al. Normothermic regional perfusion versus super rapid recovery in controlled donation after circulatory death liver transplantation. Journal of Hepatology. 2019;**70**:658-665. DOI: 10.1016/j.jhep.2018.12.013

[51] Kron P, Schlegel A, Mancina L, Clavien PA, Dutkowski P. Hypothermic oxygenated perfusion (HOPE) for fatty liver grafts in rats and humans. Journal of Hepatology. 21 Sep 2017:S0168-8278(17)32268-32267. DOI: 10.1016/j.jhep.2017.08.028. Epub ahead of print. PMID: 28870676

[52] Dutkowski P, Furrer K, Tian Y, Graf R, Clavien PA. Novel short-term hypothermic oxygenated perfusion (HOPE) system prevents injury in rat liver graft from nonheart beating donor. Annals of Surgery. 2006;**244**:968-976

[53] Guarrera JV, Henry SD, Samstein B, Odeh-Ramadan R, Kinkhabwala M, Goldstein MJ, et al. Hypothermic

machine preservation in human liver transplantation: The first clinical series. American Journal of Transplantation. 2010;**10**(2):372-381. DOI: 10.1111/j.1600-6143.2009.02932.x. Epub 2009 Dec 2

[54] van Rijn R, Karimian N, Matton APM, Burlage LC, Westerkamp AC, van den Berg AP, et al. Dual hypothermic oxygenated machine perfusion in liver transplants donated after circulatory death. The British Journal of Surgery. 2017;**104**(7):907-917. DOI: 10.1002/bjs.10515. Epub 2017 Apr 10

[55] Schlegel A, Muller X, Kalisvaart M, Muellhaupt B, Perera MTPR, Isaac JR, et al. Outcomes of DCD liver transplantation using organs treated by hypothermic oxygenated perfusion before implantation. Journal of Hepatology. 2019;**70**(1):50-57. DOI: 10.1016/j.jhep.2018.10.005. Epub 2018 Oct 18

[56] Czigany Z, Pratschke J, Froněk J, Guba M, Schöning W, Raptis DA, et al. Hypothermic oxygenated machine perfusion reduces early allograft injury and improves post-transplant outcomes in extended criteria donation liver transplantation from donation after brain death: Results from a Multicenter randomized controlled trial (HOPE ECD-DBD). Annals of Surgery. 2021;**274**(5):705-712. DOI: 10.1097/SLA.0000000000005110

[57] van Rijn R, Schurink IJ, de Vries Y, van den Berg AP, Cortes Cerisuelo M, Darwish Murad S, et al. Hypothermic machine perfusion in liver transplantation - a randomized trial. The New England Journal of Medicine. 2021;**384**(15):1391-1401. DOI: 10.1056/NEJMoa2031532. Epub 2021 Feb 24

[58] Watson CJE, Kosmoliaptsis V, Pley C, Randle L, Fear C, Crick K, et al. Observations on the ex situ perfusion of livers for transplantation. American Journal of Transplantation. 2018 Aug;**18**(8):2005-2020. DOI: 10.1111/ajt.14687. Epub 2018 Mar 14

[59] Quintini C, Del Prete L, Simioni A, Del Angel L, Diago Uso T, D'Amico G, et al. Transplantation of declined livers after normothermic perfusion. Surgery. 2022;**171**(3):747-756. DOI: 10.1016/j.surg.2021.10.056. Epub 2022 Jan 19

[60] Markmann JF, Abouljoud MS, Ghobrial RM, Bhati CS, Pelletier SJ, Lu AD, et al. Impact of portable normothermic blood-based machine perfusion on outcomes of liver transplant: The OCS liver PROTECT randomized clinical trial. JAMA Surgery. 2022;**157**(3):189-198. DOI: 10.1001/jamasurg.2021.6781

[61] Chan SC, Fan ST. Historical perspective of living donor liver transplantation. World Journal of Gastroenterology. 2008;**14**(1):15-21. DOI: 10.3748/wjg.14.15

[62] Rela M, Reddy MS. Living donor liver transplant (LDLT) is the way forward in Asia. Hepatology International. 2017;**11**(2):148-151. DOI: 10.1007/s12072-016-9780-z. Epub 2017 Jan 17

[63] Song GW, Lee SG. Living donor liver transplantation. Current Opinion in Organ Transplantation. 2014;**19**(3):217-222. DOI: 10.1097/MOT.0000000000000088

[64] Cheah YL, Simpson MA, Pomposelli JJ, Pomfret EA. Incidence of death and potentially life-threatening near-miss events in living donor hepatic lobectomy: A world-wide survey. Liver Transplantation. 2013;**19**(5):499-506. DOI: 10.1002/lt.23575

[65] Olthoff KM, Emond JC, Shearon TH, Everson G, Baker TB, Fisher RA, et al. Liver regeneration after living donor transplantation: Adult-to-adult living donor liver transplantation cohort study. Liver Transplantation. 2015;**21**(1):79-88. DOI: 10.1002/lt.23966. Epub 2014 Oct 6

[66] Ladner DP, Dew MA, Forney S, Gillespie BW, Brown RS Jr, Merion RM, et al. Long-term quality of life after liver donation in the adult to adult living donor liver transplantation cohort study (A2ALL). Journal of Hepatology. 2015;**62**(2):346-353. DOI: 10.1016/j.jhep.2014.08.043. Epub 2014 Sep 6

[67] Muzaale AD, Dagher NN, Montgomery RA, Taranto SE, McBride MA, Segev DL. Estimates of early death, acute liver failure, and long-term mortality among live liver donors. Gastroenterology. 2012;**142**(2):273-280. DOI: 10.1053/j.gastro.2011.11.015. Epub 2011 Nov 19

[68] Fan ST, Lo CM, Liu CL, et al. Safety of donors in live donor liver transplantation using right lobe grafts. Archives of Surgery. 2000;**135**:336-340

[69] Oshita A, Tashiro H, Amano H, Kobayashi T, Onoe T, Ide K, et al. Safety and feasibility of diet-treated donors with steatotic livers at the initial consultation for living-donor liver transplantation. Transplantation. 2012;**93**(10):1024-1030. DOI: 10.1097/TP.0b013e31824c9e25

[70] Organ Procurement and Transplantation Network. Available from: http://optn.transplant.hrsa.gov

[71] Onaca N, Davis GL, Goldstein RM, et al. Expanded criteria for liver transplantation in patients with hepatocellular carcinoma: A report from the international registry of hepatic tumors in liver transplantation. Liver Transplantation. 2007;**13**:391-399

[72] Nadalin S, Bockhorn M, Malagó M, Valentin-GamazoC, FrillingA, BroelschCE. Living donor liver transplantation. HPB: The Official Journal of the International Hepato Pancreato Biliary Association. 2006;**8**(1):10-21. DOI: 10.1080/13651820500465626

[73] Berg CL, Gillespie BW, Merion RM, Brown RS Jr, Abecassis MM, Trotter JF, et al. Improvement in survival associated with adult-to-adult living donor liver transplantation. Gastroenterology. 2007;**133**(6):1806-1813. DOI: 10.1053/j.gastro.2007.09.004. Epub 2007 Sep 14

[74] Olthoff KM, Merion RM, Ghobrial RM, Abecassis MM, Fair JH, Fisher RA, et al. Outcomes of 385 adult-to-adult living donor liver transplant recipients: A report from the A2ALL consortium. Annals of Surgery. 2005;**242**(3):314-323. discussion 323-5. DOI: 10.1097/01.sla.0000179646.37145.ef

[75] Berg CL, Merion RM, Shearon TH, Olthoff KM, Brown RS Jr, Baker TB, et al. Liver transplant recipient survival benefit with living donation in the model for endstage liver disease allocation era. Hepatology. 2011;**54**(4):1313-1321. DOI: 10.1002/hep.24494

[76] Goldberg DS, French B, Abt PL, Olthoff K, Shaked A. Superior survival using living donors and donor-recipient matching using a novel living donor risk index. Hepatology. 2014;**60**(5):1717-1726. DOI: 10.1002/hep.27307. Epub 2014 Oct 2

[77] Terrault NA, Shiffman ML, Lok AS, Saab S, Tong L, Brown RS Jr, et al. Outcomes in hepatitis C virus-infected recipients of living donor vs. deceased donor liver transplantation. Liver Transplantation. 2007;**13**(1):122-129. DOI: 10.1002/lt.20995

[78] Cotter TG, Minhem M, Wang J, Peeraphatdit T, Ayoub F, Pillai A, et al. Living donor liver transplantation in the United States: Evolution of frequency, outcomes, Center volumes, and factors associated with outcomes. Liver Transplantation. 2021;**27**(7):1019-1031. DOI: 10.1002/lt.26029. Epub 2021 Jun 24

Chapter 3

Extended Criteria Donors: Opportunities and Advances

Rohan M. Goswami, Kristopher Croome, Jesus Bautista and Shriya Sharma

Abstract

In recent years, remarkable advancements have been achieved in the field of liver transplantation, offering renewed hope and better outcomes for individuals with end-stage liver disease or acute liver failure who rely on orthotopic liver transplantation (OLT) as their sole treatment option. Nevertheless, the scarcity of suitable donor organs continues to present a major hurdle for patients in need of liver transplants. Tragically, the demand for donor livers surpasses the limited supply, leaving numerous patients at risk of mortality while awaiting transplantation. In response to the persistent challenge of organ donation, scientists and medical experts are actively investigating the potential of extended criteria donors (ECDs) as a potential solution. ECDs encompass a wide range of potential donors, including older individuals and those with medical conditions or viral infections, who may not meet the conventional criteria for organ acceptance.

Keywords: DCD, liver transplantation, extended criteria, end stage liver disease, cirrhosis

1. Introduction

In recent years, remarkable advancements have been achieved in the field of liver transplantation, offering renewed hope and better outcomes for individuals with end-stage liver disease or acute liver failure who rely on orthotopic liver transplantation (OLT) as their sole treatment option. Nevertheless, the scarcity of suitable donor organs continues to present a major hurdle for patients in need of liver transplants. Tragically, the demand for donor livers surpasses the limited supply, leaving numerous patients at risk of mortality while awaiting transplantation [1].

In response to the persistent challenge of organ donation, scientists and medical experts are actively investigating the potential of extended criteria donors (ECDs) as a potential solution. ECDs encompass a wide range of potential donors, including older individuals and those with medical conditions or viral infections, who may not meet the conventional criteria for organ acceptance. While a young brain-dead donor remains the preferred choice for liver transplants, exploring various other viable options for transplantation is crucial in addressing this issue (**Table 1**) [2].

Categories of extended criteria donors
Advanced donor age > 60 years
Steatosis (Macrovesicular steatosis > 30%)
Organ dysfunction at procurement • ICU stay > 7 days • Hypernatremia > 165 • Bilirubin > 3 • Elevated aspartate aminotransferase/alanine aminotransferase • Vasopressor use
Cause of death including anoxia or cerebrovascular accident
Extrahepatic malignancy
Disease transmission: HBsAg+, Hepatitis C, CDC high risk donors, HIV positive,
Long cold ischemia time (>12 h)
DCD

Table 1.
Characteristics of extended criteria donors.

A study conducted by Tector et al., has shown that the use of extended criteria donors (ECDs) has successfully addressed the shortage of suitable donor livers for transplantation, resulting in shorter wait times and improved survival. Evidence has showcased the favorable effect of utilizing extended criteria donor (ECD) livers on transplant outcomes, which are comparable to those achieved with standard donors. This highlights the potential of ECD livers as a valuable resource in addressing the critical shortage of organs, offering a promising solution to the ongoing organ shortage crisis [3].

Due to the heightened potential risks associated with different types of extended criteria donor (ECD) allografts, it is essential for medical professionals and patients to engage in a thorough discussion about the potential hazards and benefits before consenting to an organ transplant. By carefully selecting ECD liver donors and matching them with appropriate recipients, it is possible to achieve excellent survival rates and reduce wait-list mortality rates effectively. Efforts have been made to increase the availability of liver donors by using donations after circulatory death (DCD), donors who are HCV-positive and HBV-positive, HIV-positive donors and donors over the age of 60. However, livers from these donors are more susceptible to damage during transplantation, ischemia-reperfusion injury, and impaired allograft function due to prolonged cold ischemia time (CIT), which increases the risk of postoperative complications. Therefore, it is crucial to conduct thorough evaluations and carefully select ECDs to mitigate the risks associated with transplantation and maximize outcomes for those in needs [4].

2. Donation after circulatory death (DCD)

The donation after circulatory death (DCD) is a process that focuses on cardiopulmonary criteria rather than neurologic criteria. It involves recovering organs for transplantation after death has been confirmed using circulatory criteria. This method differs significantly from the conventional standard model for deceased donation, which relies on the confirmation of death using neurological criteria. There is also a variable period of warm ischemia that follows before the organs can be preserved for donation. This is why DCD is often considered an ECD.

Donation after circulatory death (DCD) donor livers are divided into five categories according to modified Maastricht's classification. Categories I, II, and V pertain to the recovery of organs after an unforeseen and irreversible cardiac arrest (uncontrolled donation after circulatory death—DCD), while categories III and IV refer to the retrieval of organs after planned withdrawal of life-sustaining cardiorespiratory support (controlled DCD). Uncontrolled DCD can only take place in facilities equipped with organ perfusion and retrieval capabilities readily available, typically located near or within a transplantation center. On the other hand, controlled DCD can be supported in almost any intensive care unit (ICU) or emergency department (ED) [5].

According to the annual report from the US Organ Procurement and Transplantation Network, 10.6% of liver donations come from DCD donors unlike organs from donors who have experienced brain death [6].

A study conducted by Mihaylov et al., reviewed 135 consecutive DCD LTs and found that optimizing perioperative conditions by using a thrombolytic donor flush and minimizing ischemia times can improve outcomes for ECD DCD LT. They observed a significantly lower incidence of ischemic cholangiopathy (IC) (5% versus 17% in era 1; P = 0.03) and better 1-year graft survival (93% versus 75% in era 1; P = 0.07). This suggests that ECD DCD livers can be successfully transplanted optimizing perioperative conditions, expanding the donor pool for LT [7].

A recent study led by Duan et al. examined 1104 cases of deceased donor liver transplants, of which 807 patients received a liver from a donor after cardiac death (DCD). The researchers conducted a thorough evaluation of various donor characteristics, including age and fatty liver status. The analysis revealed that there were no significant differences in postoperative complications between the DCD and other groups, and the survival rates of both patients and grafts were similar at 90 days, 1 year, and 3 years. This study demonstrates that moderately steatotic livers from DCD donors can effectively broaden the pool of available livers for transplantation, offering valuable insights into the impact of these extended criteria on liver transplant outcomes [8].

Research shows that medical facilities with a high number of liver transplants tend to use donation after circulatory death (DCD) more frequently (over 5 times a year) than low-volume centers. This increased use of DCD is associated with better outcomes for patients, including graft survival, 1-year patient mortality, 1-year graft failure, and long-term patient survival [9]. Other study conducted by Pescarissi et al., concludes that there is potential to increase the supply and use of ECDs for transplantation and that the perioperative period of LT from selected DCD donors can be safe with careful management by experienced anesthesiologists and intensivists [10].

There is a lot of concern around post-transplantation outcomes when it comes to marginal organs. DCD livers in particular have a high rate of biliary strictures due to the period of warm ischemia between withdrawal of donor life support and organ preservation. This can lead to lower graft survival rates, increase re-transplantation, and higher hospital costs [11].

In liver transplantation, Donation after Circulatory Death (DCD) grafts are frequently utilized. These grafts, however, come with an elevated risk due to an additional ischemic event during the Donor Warm Ischemia Time (DWIT), leading to an increased chance of severe ischemia/reperfusion injury and postoperative complications like ischemic cholangiopathy. The duration of actual ischemia during DWIT varies widely among donors and depends on the course of vital parameters after life support withdrawal. This ischemic period, known as the functional DWIT, begins when either Spo2 (oxygen saturation) or blood pressure drops below a certain threshold and continues until the commencement of cold perfusion during organ retrieval. Numerous retrospective single and multicenter studies have examined the impact of DWIT on liver transplantation outcomes. However, there is still no standardized definition for DWIT, leading to the incorporation of different definitions and classifications by various authors to better understand its dynamics. Developing a unified definition for DWIT could aid clinicians in optimizing the utilization of DCD livers and reducing the risk of complications [12].

A liver transplantation (LT) using donation after circulatory death (DCD) has seen progress, but ischemic cholangiopathy (IC) remains a concern. IC is the primary cause of DCD graft loss and has prevented many transplant centers from accepting DCD grafts. Despite extensive research, the cause of IC is still unclear.

A study by Goussous et al. analyzed 112 patients who underwent liver transplantation from DCD between 2005 and 2017. In 2014, measures were taken to reduce donor hepatectomy time (DHT) and cold ischemic time (CIT) to improve DCD LT outcomes. The group that received transplants after the changes had shorter DHT and CIT, and fewer cases of IC than the historical group [13].

In a meta-analysis conducted by Jay et al., a comparison of biliary complications after liver transplantation was undertaken. The study examined 489 transplants from DCD donors and 4455 transplants from DBD donors. The findings indicated that DCD recipients had a higher overall rate of biliary complications (29%) compared to DBD recipients (17%). Specifically, DCD recipients had 2.4 times greater odds of experiencing biliary complications than those who received DBD transplants. Moreover, the study revealed that DCD recipients had a higher incidence of ischemic cholangiopathy (IC) (16%) compared to DBD recipients (3%), with DCD recipients having 10.8 times greater odds of developing IC [14].

In a recent study conducted by Mercado et al., the impact of portal vein thrombosis (PVT) during liver transplantation (LT) from donation after circulatory death (DCD) donors was investigated. The study revealed that PVT can add complexity to the surgical procedure. However, carefully selected recipients with grades I-II PVT showed successful outcomes when receiving DCD liver grafts. There were no significant differences in outcomes between patients with or without PVT with grades I-II, including rates of early allograft dysfunction, primary nonfunction, or ischemic cholangiopathy [15].

Also, according to Black et al. in 2022, living donor liver transplantation (LDLT) provides superior 5-year patient and graft survival rates compared to deceased donor liver transplantation (DCD-LT). LDLT also has comparable outcomes to deceased brain-dead donor liver transplantation (DBD-LT) in terms of survival rates, but it has a higher rate of readmissions. Despite this, LDLT has a higher rate of return to work and a lower rate of chronic kidney disease (CKD). When possible, LDLT should be the preferred method over DCD-LT. However, increasing the utilization of both LDLT and DCD-LT can help more patients gain access to life-saving liver transplants [16].

A recent study conducted by Haque et al. analyzed data from 33,429 deceased-donor liver transplants in the US from 2002 to 2008. The study followed up for 10 years after the implementation of MELD and compared transplantation outcomes between recipients of donation after circulatory death (DCD) and donation after brain death (DBD). The results showed that while DCD had lower 10-year graft survival compared to DBD, the rates of graft failure for both groups were the same after the first year post-transplant. Moreover, patient survival was similar between the two groups. The study suggests that the use of DCD livers could increase with the development of machine perfusion technology to address early biliary complications [17].

Donation after circulatory death (DCD) liver transplant recipients have experienced worse survival rates compared to DBD recipients due to the inevitable WIT during the declaration of death and organ retrieval process. To improve DCD liver transplant outcomes, multiple interventions have been suggested to recondition DCD liver grafts. Interventions, before and after death, may increase the likelihood of organs being suitable for transplant. Research has shown that pharmacologic protection and machine perfusion of the liver are promising strategies to protect against ischemia-reperfusion injury, especially for high-risk organs. These strategies aim to improve the viability and number of organs available for transplant and increase the likelihood of organs being suitable, ultimately expanding the donor pool. Also, liver transplants using cold preservation methods often lead to ischemia-reperfusion injury (IRI) in the donor's liver. Donor livers that undergo normothermic machine perfusion (NMP) are also susceptible to IRI. NMP mimics the physiologic liver perfusion by utilizing a red blood cell-based solution at temperatures between 35.5 and 37.5°C, offering a range of potential benefits. The potential effects of normothermic perfusion include countering hyperfibrinolysis and inflammation after reperfusion, replenishing glycogen, and promoting the regeneration of adenosine triphosphate. Studies on normothermic machine perfusion are centered around developing biomarkers to predict allograft quality and susceptibility to ischemia-reperfusion injury. Additionally, normothermic perfusion of marginal allografts allows for the implementation of various therapeutic interventions to potentially enhance organ quality. Based on current clinical trials, normothermic perfusion not only increases the utilization of hepatic allografts but also appears to be associated with milder ischemia-reperfusion injury, leading to a reduced risk of early allograft dysfunction and fewer biliary complications, including ischemic cholangiopathy, compared to static cold storage [18].

Normothermic regional perfusion (NRP) is a method used to maintain allografts obtained from DCD by employing VA-ECMO to sustain thoracic and abdominal organ perfusion, allowing time for recovery from warm ischemic injury. Two forms of NRP are currently in use, depending on the organ being procured. Thoracoabdominal NRP (TA-NRP) for donors with planned heart and abdominal organ recovery, and abdominal NRP (A-NRP) for donors with only abdominal organ recovery. NRP offers several advantages, including continuous warm blood perfusion, which aids in restoring heart function, reducing myocardial injury, and maintaining organ homeostasis. It allows visual assessment of organs, promotes organ recovery by establishing perfusion, reduces warm ischemia time, and enables viability assessment in a non-ischemic state before retrieval, unlike direct cold storage. Limiting factors for broad application of NRP are related to implementation and acceptance by organ procurement organizations. The process of NRP is complex, requiring coordination among donor hospitals, procurement teams, perfusionists, and organ procurement organizations, with successful execution contingent upon agreement from all involved parties [19].

3. Donors of advanced age

The age range of liver donors for transplantation has changed significantly in recent years. The United Network for Organ Sharing (UNOS) reported that in 1989, only 2.4% of donors were above 50 years old. However, by 2013, this number had increased to 33%. In the past, donating a liver after 50 was not recommended as it was believed to be associated with poor outcomes. But recent studies have shown that older donors without additional risk factors can have results similar to younger donors [20].

The liver is more resistant to aging in healthy individuals compared to other organs because it has a large functional reserve, dual blood supply that exceeds its metabolic needs, and regenerative capacity. However, as livers from older donors are smaller in weight and volume and may have developed fibrous thickening of the capsule, it is unclear if these changes affect organ function after transplantation [21, 22].

The outcomes of liver transplants from donors over the age of 70 were examined in a study by Alamo et al. they found that while survival rates were similar, there was a greater incidence of ascites and primary dysfunction due to delayed graft function. Certain factors such as the recipient's Model for End-Stage Liver Disease (MELD) score, cold ischemia time, diabetes, hypertension, and weight over 90 kg were associated with poor prognosis. The study concluded that liver transplants from elderly donors are safe, but careful selection of both donors and recipients is necessary [23].

Another study by Kim et al. analyzed liver transplant outcomes from donors aged 65 years and above and identified several factors that affected graft survival. They found that older donor livers should not be dismissed solely based on age and that they can result in good graft survival in selected cases [24].

Wang et al., divided 159 patients into two groups based on donor age and found no significant differences in graft or recipient survival rates at 1, 3, and 5 years. However, the older donor group required a larger volume of red blood cell transfusions during the surgical procedure. The authors concluded that Liver transplant with donors older than 50 years is safe and does not have significant adverse effects on graft function or long-term donor and patient survival [25].

Although the age of the liver donor is an important factor in liver transplantation outcomes, it is not the only factor to consider. Other factors such as surgical conditions, including ischemia time and hemodynamic instability during surgery, as well as recipient conditions, such as MELD score, also play a crucial role. Therefore, minimizing these Liver transplants with elderly donors can have similar outcomes to those with younger donors. Accepting an old liver donor (OLD) graft can improve survival for all waitlist candidates, especially those with high MELD scores. It's important to note that both older and younger candidates benefit from accepting an OLD graft. Patients and providers should carefully consider the consequences of declining an OLD graft offer, as a quarter of candidates die after such a decline. These findings can help transplant providers make better decisions and improve patient counseling. Another consideration with aged donors is the risk of transmitting malignancy due to the higher incidence of unrecognized malignancies in the elderly [26].

4. Donors with viral infections

Viruses such as Hepatitis B and Hepatitis C are routinely screened in potential donors due to their potential impact. However, these infections can be managed effectively, especially in individuals with weakened immune systems. Therefore, a positive test result for these viruses does not necessarily disqualify someone from being a suitable donor.

4.1 Hepatitis B virus (HBV)

The prevalence of hepatitis B core antibody (HBcAb) positivity varies across different geographic locations. In liver donors within the United States, the prevalence is reported to be 4.8%. Considering the global prevalence of HBV "past" and present infections, with 2 billion and 350 million affected individuals respectively, the use of liver grafts from donors with past HBV infection (HBcAb-positive only) is a relatively common practice. This approach holds the potential to significantly alleviate the shortage of organs, especially in countries with high HBV endemicity. However, it is essential to note that donors who test positive for HBcAb may carry intrahepatic covalently closed circular DNA (cDNA) and may also have an occult infection with positive serum HBV DNA [27].

Donors who are hepatitis B surface antigen negative (HBsAg−) but hepatitis B core antigen positive (anti-HBc+) have transmitted HBV infection to liver recipients who are HBsAg−. Early studies of the use of hepatitis B core antibody-positive allografts to treat HBV+ recipients suggested that the risk of HBV transmission was extremely high and carried high mortality. However, in patients who are immune to HBV (previous vaccination), it is safe to use these organs [28]. Additionally, donors with positive hepatitis B surface antibodies (anti-HBs) do not appear to transmit HBV infection after liver transplantation.

The use of combined prophylaxis with hepatitis B immune globulin (HBIg) and lamivudine has proven effective against HBV recurrence and de-novo HBV infection or transmission in recipients of anti-HBcAb+ livers [29, 30].

Further data has shown that using an HBsAg-positive graft is feasible. HBsAg-positive recipients who received a graft from HBsAg-positive inactive carriers remained HBsAg positive, and HBIg was discontinued within the first-month post-LT. This experience demonstrates that LT using grafts from deceased HBsAg-positive donors is feasible and may expand the pool of organ donors with appropriate antiviral management and monitoring [31].

In a study by Saidi et al., the United Network for Organ Sharing (UNOS) database was used to review LT outcome data in the United States. The study found that both the graft and the patient had similar survival rates between the 92 recipients of HBsAg-positive grafts and recipients of HBsAg-negative grafts. The majority of the study population required LT for HBV-related disease (74%) [32].

The largest series describing the transplantation of HBV NAT+ kidney and liver allografts aimed to assess the 1-year safety and effectiveness of such transplants in seronegative kidney transplant (KT) and liver transplant (LT) recipients. Over a 1-year period, 89 recipients received HBV NAT+ organs, and no HBV-related complications were observed. Among 18 recipients who experienced viremic episodes, 16 of them achieved undetectable HBV DNA levels after approximately 80 days of entecavir therapy. Expanding the use of HBV NAT+ organs in nonviremic recipients may help alleviate the national organ shortage [33].

4.2 Hepatitis C virus (HCV)

In the past, there was much debate about using organs from donors with Hepatitis C virus (HCV+) for liver transplantation (LT). However, due to a shortage of organs for transplant, the use of HCV+ organs has become more common as a solution to increase the donor pool. Despite advances in treatment, many HCV+ liver allografts, several hundred per year, are still not being used. HCV infection affects an estimated 1–2% of the general US population, but the risk is higher (3–18%) among organ donors with more risk factors as defined by the Public Health Service [34].

A study by Alvaro et al. found that using HCV+ donors is a safe and effective source for liver donation. Out of 143 transplants performed in HCV+ recipients, 9.1% received an organ from an anti-HCV+ donor, with 72.7% showing a negative viral load. Although 80% of the patients experienced hepatitis during follow-up, there was no significant difference in patient or graft survival observed between the two groups [35].

A retrospective study by Ting et al. demonstrated that HCV seronegative patients who receive an HCV seropositive liver allograft can have good short-term outcomes with HCV cure following antiviral treatment [36].

Evaluating long-term outcomes in liver transplant recipients transplanted with HCV antibody-positive organs, A study conducted by Stepanova et al., in 2016 evaluated the long-term outcomes of liver transplant recipients who received organs from donors with HCV antibodies. The study compared the rates of mortality and graft loss between those who received organs from HCV antibody-positive (HCV+) donors and those who received organs from HCV antibody-negative donors. The study found that both mortality rates and graft loss rates were similar between HCV patients transplanted from HCV+ donors and those transplanted from HCV-negative donors. In fact, long-term outcomes were very similar in patients who received organs from HCV+ and HCV− donors [37].

A cross-sectional study by Da et al., found that HCV-positive donors were healthier and donated superior liver allografts compared with HCV-negative donors. The use of an HCV donor is a good option to increase the organ pool. Several studies suggest that LT from HCV+ donors are a safe procedure with the use of effective antiviral therapy [38].

4.3 Human immunodeficiency virus (HIV)

The worldwide occurrence of human immunodeficiency virus (HIV) has now affected 37 million people. Although antiretroviral treatment has been developed, HIV-unrelated reasons have become significant factors in determining survival rates. Liver disease is one of the main causes of death, accounting for 10%. This rise in prevalence is because of the high frequency of concomitant HBV and HCV infections with HIV. Consequently, it is crucial to encourage organ transplantation in this population, as HIV-infected recipients have similar survival rates to non-infected recipients, albeit with three times higher acute rejection rates [39]. Currently, organs from HIV-positive donors can only be transplanted to HIV-positive patients. In nations with a high prevalence of HIV, liver transplantation from HIV-positive donors has become a desirable choice. Furthermore, almost 66% of HIV-positive individuals are eager to donate their organs to other HIV-positive patients. They have distinct reasons, such as combating HIV-related prejudices and showing compassion toward other infected patients [40]. According to a recent publication by Rozera et al., it has been confirmed that HIV-positive individuals can safely receive transplants from HIV-positive donors without the risk of superinfection. The immunosuppressive treatment administered to prevent transplant rejection does not seem to have a significant impact on the progression of HIV disease or any other viral reactivations [41].

5. Conclusion

This chapter provides comprehensive insights into various aspects of liver transplantation, focusing on the utilization of extended criteria donors- including those from donation after circulatory death and donors with viral infections such as hepatitis B and hepatitis C. The findings emphasize the importance of expanding the donor pool to address the critical shortage of organs for transplantation. Despite the potential risks associated with ECDs, studies demonstrate promising outcomes with careful selection and optimization of perioperative conditions. Advancements in antiviral therapy and transplant management contribute to improved survival rates and outcomes for recipients of ECD livers, highlighting the significance of ongoing research and innovation in liver transplantation. Further studies are warranted to continue refining strategies for donor selection, perioperative management, and long-term outcomes, ultimately enhancing the effectiveness and accessibility of liver transplantation for patients in need.

Author details

Rohan M. Goswami*, Kristopher Croome, Jesus Bautista and Shriya Sharma
Mayo Clinic, Florida, USA

*Address all correspondence to: goswami.rohan@mayo.edu

References

[1] Vodkin I, Kuo A. Extended criteria donors in liver transplantation. Clinics in Liver Disease. 2017;**21**(2):289-301. DOI: 10.1016/j.cld.2016.12.004

[2] Nair A, Hashimoto K. Extended criteria donors in liver transplantation-from marginality to mainstream. Hepatobiliary Surgery and Nutrition. 2018;**7**(5):386-388. DOI: 10.21037/hbsn.2018.06.08

[3] Tector AJ et al. Use of extended criteria livers decreases wait time for liver transplantation without adversely impacting post-transplant survival. Annals of Surgery. 2006;**244**(3):439-450. DOI: 10.1097/01.sla.0000234896.18207.fa

[4] Nostedt JJ et al. Addressing organ shortages: Progress in donation after circulatory death for liver transplantation. Canadian Journal of Surgery. Journal Canadien de Chirurgie. 2020;**63**(2):E135-E141. DOI: 10.1503/cjs.005519

[5] Manara AR et al. Donation after circulatory death. British Journal of Anaesthesia. 2012;**108**(Suppl. 1):i108-i121. DOI: 10.1093/bja/aer357

[6] Annual data report of the US organ procurement and transplantation network. Preface. American Journal of Transplantation: Official Journal of the American Society of Transplantation and the American Society of Transplant Surgeons. 2014;**14**(Suppl. 1):5-7. DOI: 10.1111/ajt.12626

[7] Mihaylov P et al. Expanding the donor pool with the use of extended criteria donation after circulatory death livers. Liver Transplantation: Official Publication of the American Association for the Study of Liver Diseases and the International Liver Transplantation Society. 2019;**25**(8):1198-1208. DOI: 10.1002/lt.25462

[8] Duan X et al. Outcomes of liver transplantation using moderately steatotic liver from donation after cardiac death (DCD). Annals of Translational Medicine. 2020;**8**(18):1188. DOI: 10.21037/atm-20-5888

[9] Delman AM et al. The volume-outcomes relationship in donation after circulatory death liver transplantation. Clinical Transplantation. 2022;**36**(6):e14658. DOI: 10.1111/ctr.14658

[10] Pescarissi C et al. The perioperative period of liver transplantation from unconventional extended criteria donors: Data from two high-volume centres. BMC Anesthesiology. 2022;**22**(1):390. DOI: 10.1186/s12871-022-01932-x

[11] Axelrod DA et al. The economic impact of the utilization of liver allografts with high donor risk index. American Journal of Transplantation: Official Journal of the American Society of Transplantation and the American Society of Transplant Surgeons. 2007;**7**(4):990-997. DOI: 10.1111/j.1600-6143.2006.01724.x

[12] Kalisvaart M et al. Donor warm ischemia time in DCD liver transplantation-working group report from the ILTS DCD, liver preservation, and machine perfusion consensus conference. Transplantation. 2021;**105**(6):1156-1164. DOI: 10.1097/TP.0000000000003819

[13] Goussous N et al. Ischemic cholangiopathy postdonation after circulatory death liver transplantation:

Donor hepatectomy time matters. Transplantation Direct. 2021;**8**(1):e1277. DOI: 10.1097/TXD.0000000000001277

[14] Jay CL et al. Ischemic cholangiopathy after controlled donation after cardiac death liver transplantation: A meta-analysis. Annals of Surgery. 2011;**253**(2):259-264. DOI: 10.1097/SLA.0b013e318204e658

[15] Mercado LA et al. DCD liver grafts can safely be used for recipients with grade I-II portal vein thrombosis: A multicenter analysis. Transplantation Direct. 2022;**8**(11):e1392. DOI: 10.1097/TXD.0000000000001392

[16] Black M et al. Living donor liver transplantation versus donation after brain death and donation after circulatory death liver transplantation in the US. Proceedings (Baylor University. Medical Center). 2022;**35**(3):273-277. DOI: 10.1080/08998280.2022.2034202

[17] Haque OJ et al. Long-term outcomes of early experience in donation after circulatory death liver transplantation: Outcomes at 10 years. Annals of Transplantation. 2021;**26**:e930243. DOI: 10.12659/AOT.930243

[18] van Beekum CJ et al. Normothermic machine perfusion (NMP) of the liver-current status and future perspectives. Annals of Transplantation. 2021;**26**:e931664. DOI: 10.12659/AOT.931664

[19] Alamouti-Fard E et al. Normothermic regional perfusion is an emerging cost-effective alternative in donation after circulatory death (DCD) in heart transplantation. Cureus. 2022;**14**(6):e26437. DOI: 10.7759/cureus.26437

[20] Grazi GL et al. A revised consideration on the use of very aged donors for liver transplantation. American Journal of Transplantation: Official Journal of the American Society of Transplantation and the American Society of Transplant Surgeons. 2001;**1**(1):61-68. DOI: 10.1034/j.1600-6143.2001.010112.x

[21] Sersté T, Bourgeois N. Ageing and the liver. Acta Gastro-Enterologica Belgica. 2006;**69**(3):296-298

[22] Durand F et al. Age and liver transplantation. Journal of Hepatology. 2019;**70**(4):745-758. DOI: 10.1016/j.jhep.2018.12.009

[23] Alamo J-M et al. Donor characteristics that are associated with survival in liver transplant recipients older than 70 years with grafts. Transplantation Proceedings. 2013;**45**(10):3633-3636. DOI: 10.1016/j.transproceed.2013.10.031

[24] Kim DY et al. Liver transplantation using elderly donors: A risk factor analysis. Clinical Transplantation. 2011;**25**(2):270-276. DOI: 10.1111/j.1399-0012.2010.01222.x

[25] Wang K et al. Effect of donor age on graft function and long-term survival of recipients undergoing living donor liver transplantation. Hepatobiliary & Pancreatic Diseases International: HBPD INT. 2015;**14**(1):50-55. DOI: 10.1016/s1499-3872(15)60334-4

[26] Hashimoto K, Miller C. The use of marginal grafts in liver transplantation. Journal of Hepato-Biliary-Pancreatic Surgery. 2008;**15**(2):92-101. DOI: 10.1007/s00534-007-1300-z

[27] Cholongitas E et al. Liver grafts from anti-hepatitis B core positive donors: A systematic review. Journal of Hepatology. 2010;**52**(2):272-279. DOI: 10.1016/j.jhep.2009.11.009

[28] Hou X et al. Current status and recent advances in liver transplant using organs donated after cardiac death. Experimental and Clinical Transplantation: Official Journal of the Middle East Society for Organ Transplantation. 2015;**13**(1):6-18

[29] Ho JK et al. Utilization of a liver allograft from a hepatitis B surface antigen positive donor. Transplantation. 2006;**81**(1):129-131. DOI: 10.1097/01.tp.0000191946.49884.40

[30] Gane EJ et al. Lamivudine plus low-dose hepatitis B immunoglobulin to prevent recurrent hepatitis B following liver transplantation. Gastroenterology. 2007;**132**(3):931-937. DOI: 10.1053/j.gastro.2007.01.005

[31] Choi YR et al. Liver transplantation for HBsAg-positive recipients using grafts from HBsAg-positive deceased donors. Transplant International: Official Journal of the European Society for Organ Transplantation. 2013;**26**(12):1173-1183. DOI: 10.1111/tri.12177

[32] Saidi RF et al. Liver transplantation from hepatitis B surface antigen-positive donors. Transplantation Proceedings. 2013;**45**(1):279-280. DOI: 10.1016/j.transproceed.2012.05.077

[33] Delman AM et al. Expanding the donor pool: First use of hepatitis B virus nat positive solid organ allografts into seronegative recipients. Annals of Surgery. 2021;**274**(4):556-564. DOI: 10.1097/SLA.0000000000005071

[34] Ellingson K et al. Estimated risk of human immunodeficiency virus and hepatitis C virus infection among potential organ donors from 17 organ procurement organizations in the United States. American Journal of Transplantation: Official Journal of the American Society of Transplantation and the American Society of Transplant Surgeons. 2011;**11**(6):1201-1208. DOI: 10.1111/j.1600-6143.2011.03518.x

[35] Álvaro E et al. Liver transplantation from anti-hepatitis C virus-positive donors: Our experience. Transplantation Proceedings. 2012;**44**(6):1475-1478. DOI: 10.1016/j.transproceed.2012.05.012

[36] Ting P-S et al. Hepatitis C-positive donor liver transplantation for hepatitis C seronegative recipients. Transplant Infectious Disease: An Official Journal of the Transplantation Society. 2019;**21**(6):e13194. DOI: 10.1111/tid.13194

[37] Stepanova M, Sayiner M, de Avila L, Younoszai Z, Racila A, Younossi ZM. Long-term outcomes of liver transplantation in patients with hepatitis C infection are not affected by HCV positivity of a donor. BMC Gastroenterology. 2016;**16**(1):137. DOI: 10.1186/s12876-016-0551-z

[38] Da BL, Ezaz G, Kushner T, Crismale J, Kakked G, Gurakar A, et al. Donor characteristics and regional differences in the utilization of HCV-positive donors in liver transplantation. JAMA Network Open. 2020;**3**(12):e2027551. DOI: 10.1001/jamanetworkopen.2020.27551

[39] Werbel WA, Durand CM. Solid organ transplantation in HIV-infected recipients: History, progress, and frontiers. Current HIV/AIDS Reports. 2019;**16**(3):191-203. DOI: 10.1007/s11904-019-00440-x

[40] Rasmussen VP, Sarah E, et al. Perceptions, motivations, and concerns about living organ donation among people living with HIV. AIDS Care. 2018;**30**(12):1595-1599. DOI: 10.1080/09540121.2018.1469724

[41] Rozera G et al. Analysis of HIV quasispecies and virological outcome of an HIV D+/R+ kidney-liver transplantation. Virology Journal. 2022;**19**(1):4. DOI: 10.1186/s12985-021-01730-w

Section 3

The Future of Liver Transplantation

Chapter 4

Dd-cfDNA in Liver Transplantation: The Future of Non-Invasive Liver Graft Evaluation

Eleni Avramidou, Stella Vasileiadou and Georgios Tsoulfas

Abstract

Donor-derived cell-free DNA (Dd-cfDNA) is a novel biomarker with many diagnostic applications in various areas of medicine and particularly transplantation. This biomarker is derived from donor cells that have undergone apoptosis or cell death and thus reflects possible graft damage. Regarding the field of liver transplantation, dd-cfDNA can contribute to the diagnosis of complications that include signs of rejection or other types of possible graft injury. Measurements of dd-cfDNA also depend on the graft's size and origin; therefore, these data should be considered for the estimation and explanation of dd-cfDNA values. Despite the utility of this novel diagnostic technique, it comes with some limitations and application exclusions, such as cases where there is a blood relation between the donor and recipient. Combination of dd-cfDNA evaluation with the assessment of other currently used biomarkers, such as liver enzymes, or other novel biomarkers can result to high diagnostic value.

Keywords: liver transplantation, non-invasive, biomarkers, dd-cfDNA, evaluation of liver graft

1. Introduction

Liver transplantation (LT) is the only treatment option for end-stage liver failure and the best option for some specific cases of liver cancer. In 1963, Starzl et al. performed the first liver transplantation [1]. It took over a decade for LT to overcome the challenges associated with the immune response, with a noteworthy breakthrough being the application of cyclosporine, yielding positive long-term outcomes for patients [2]. Despite a steady increase in the number of LT operations with nowadays more than 35,000 liver transplants being performed globally, long-term survival beyond the first year after LT has not significantly improved in the past decades due to many factors, including the long-term effects of immunosuppression and graft dysfunction [3].

A significant obstacle to LT long-term graft and patient's survival is the lack of a reliable and non-invasive biomarker that monitors graft function and detects graft injury early. Reliable, non-invasive detection of possible damage of liver graft constitutes a prominent area of research in transplantation, with various biomarkers and biomarker panels already being researched about their specificity and sensitivity.

In this chapter, we aimed to describe the possible role of donor-derived cell-free DNA (dd-cfDNA) in the evaluation of liver graft and monitoring of liver transplant recipients.

2. Liver histology

Liver is a parenchymal organ, covered by a peritoneal lining consisting of a single-layer mesothelium disposed on a thin layer of sub-mesothelial connective tissue [4]. Regarding the morphology of the liver, this is based on morpho-functional units called hepatic lobules [5]. Each hepatic lobule appears as an area of polygonal shape, made up of laminae of epithelial cells, the hepatocytes. In the spaces between the hepatocytes, there is a dense vascular network consisting of capillaries called hepatic sinusoids. In the center of the lobule, there is a central (centrilobular) vein, while in the periphery, there are terminal branches of the portal vein and of the hepatic artery, which in combination of branches of bile ducts, they form the portal or porto-biliary spaces. Apart from this morphology model, there are some other ones proposed like the portal lobule and hepatic acinus [6]. Concerning the cell types that consist liver histology, those apart from hepatocytes include endothelial cells, hepatic stellate cells, Kupffer cells, lymphocytes, and cholangiocytes, which consist the intrahepatic bile ducts [7–10].

3. Pathophysiology of LT-related pathologies

There are many pathologies related to liver transplantation that may result in dysfunction or even non-function of the graft. These pathologies include subclinical graft injury, chronic or acute rejection, infections, and cancer. For the accurate, non-invasive diagnosis of those pathologies, a background knowledge of their pathophysiology is needed.

The most common pathology that occurs in LT and the base of other LT-related pathologies as well is the graft injury. Graft injury can be caused by ischemia-reperfusion process, with the anoxia occurring in liver tissue resulting in the generation of reactive oxygen species and initiation of a cellular cascade leading to inflammation and cell death. Apart from cell cascade and oxygen free radicals, T cells and Kupffer cells have found to be in the center of liver graft injury resulting in the observed in surveillance liver graft biopsies (svLBxs) neutrophil inflammation [11–13].

Rejection is also considered a form of graft injury with liver dysfunction being observed as well. There are two major types of rejection classified based on the time of occurrence: acute and chronic. Moreover, rejection types can be classified based on the pathophysiology mechanism on T-cell (TCR) and antibody-mediated (AMR). TCR usually occurs early, and the diagnosis is based on biopsy findings including dense portal-based mixed inflammatory cell infiltrate with the evidence of damage to biliary epithelium, portal and hepatic vein endothelium, and hepatocytes [14]. During liver inflammation, the expression of MHC class I is increased in all cell types, instead of being limited to Kupffer cells like in the normal liver, and MHC class II expression is stimulated in endothelium, biliary epithelium, and hepatocytes. Activated donor-derived dendritic cells arriving in the lymph node act as a potent immunological stimulus for recipient-derived naive CD4+ T cells. CD8+ and CD4+ T cells are participating in rejection pathophysiology by differentiating into different T-cell subtypes, primarily polarized toward the Th1 response with the secretion of many cytokines. AMR can happen early and later on, with the most severe form being the hyperacute rejection that occurs in ABO-incompatible grafts [15]. In AMR, donor-specific antibodies (DSA) play a pivotal role. They can be preformed or de novo produced by the interaction of B cells with alloantigens [16].

LT recipients are also prone to different infections due to their immunosuppressive treatment scheme. Viral infections of the liver graft like cytomegalovirus (CMV), EBV, and HCV can result in various pathophysiological alterations and dysfunction. CMV infection has a high prevalence in the general population and can be serious in recipients who were seronegative prior to liver transplantation. The pathophysiology of liver damage in CMV infections is based both on the direct effect of the virus in mesenchymal and endothelial cells and to the modulation of the immune system that may result to acute early allograft rejection or late allograft dysfunction [17]. HCV infection can be acute or chronic and, apart from immediate immune alterations, can result in liver fibrosis [18, 19].

Cancer is a very serious, rare complication of chronic immunosuppression. Apart from the rare occurrence of cancer as a result of immunosuppression, LT recipients operated for hepatocellular carcinoma (HCC) based on Milan criteria show a risk of recurrence in 8–20% of the cases [20, 21]. HCC is a highly heterogeneous cancer, both at the molecular and histological level. There is a strong correlation between HCC with fibrosis, molecular mechanisms related to comprise telomere maintenance, Wnt/β-catenin signaling and cell cycle regulation, TERT promoter alterations, and CTNNB1 and TP53 mutations [22].

4. Current methods of liver graft evaluation

In today's clinical practice, the established everyday clinical practice for graft evaluation includes the serum measurement of alanine aminotransferase (ALT) and aspartate aminotransferase (AST), along with the performance of surveillance liver graft biopsy (svLBxs). Each of those methods of evaluation is not optimal and opposes certain limitations. Particularly, for the liver function enzymes evaluation, main limitations include their lack of liver specificity, the reflection of damage of specific cell types (hepatocytes or cholangiocytes), and their long half-lives [23, 24]. Regarding svLBxs, despite its specificity in detecting and diagnosing different graft injuries and pathologies, when considering the complexity and large size of the liver, its sensitivity is far from 100%, which often leads to inaccurate diagnosis. Moreover, it remains an invasive procedure with certain risks for the patient and a high cost, all of the above leading to this not being an evidence-based applied procedure to most of the liver transplantation centers [25].

5. Recent breakthroughs in non-invasive liver graft evaluation

In recent years, precision medicine research is focused on unraveling the molecular pathways associated with specific liver graft pathologies [26]. A primary objective of this field of research is the investigation of the potential role of liver-specific biomarkers in the non-invasive accurate diagnosis. For a biomarker to be considered suitable for everyday clinical practice application, it has to fulfill certain qualifications. These include the non-invasive detection, the specificity about liver graft and sensitivity about different pathologies. Shorter half-life time and cost effectiveness are also desirable characteristics of a possible biomarker [27, 28]. There has already been found a correlation between graft dysfunction, pathologies, and different types of biomarkers including nucleic and protein ones, metabolites, and the recently discovered extracellular vesicles [29–31]. Among protein biomarkers are those involved in immune responses, like in complement system activation (C3a, C5a, and sC5b-9), C-reactive Protein, cytokines, MHC class I polypeptides, and different types of CD blood cells, enzymes such as ATP citrate lyase, apolipoprotein A1, and butyrylcholinesterase, structural proteins such as fibrinogen alpha chain, and signaling proteins such as VEGF [32–36]. The majority of the research although so far is focused on nucleic biomarkers which include different types of miRNAs, mRNAs, long non-coding RNAs(lncRNAs), DNAs, and dd-cfDNA [37–42].

6. Role of dd-cfDNA

dd-cfDNA has emerged as a non-invasive, precise biomarker for monitoring liver transplant recipients by many researchers. Over the past few years, the utilization of dd-cfDNA has witnessed a notable increase, with potential applications including the early detection of cancer and graft dysfunction in various types of transplantation [43]. Dd-cfDNA was first used by Sigdel et al. as a rapid non-invasive assay for the detection of renal transplant injury [44]. Originating from apoptotic cells within the graft, dd-cfDNA exhibits remarkable specificity, with a limitation in sensitivity. Dd-cfDNA has applications in every type of solid organ transplantation, a characteristic that justifies the extensive research existing about this emerging biomarker [45].

7. Methods of evaluation of dd-cfDNA

Dd-cfDNA is measured most usually in serum or in plasma and sometimes in urine, especially when it comes to kidney transplantation monitoring [46]. Its assessment includes an evaluation of its quantity, but also an investigation of some quality characteristics, such as the size of the fragments and methylation patterns [47].

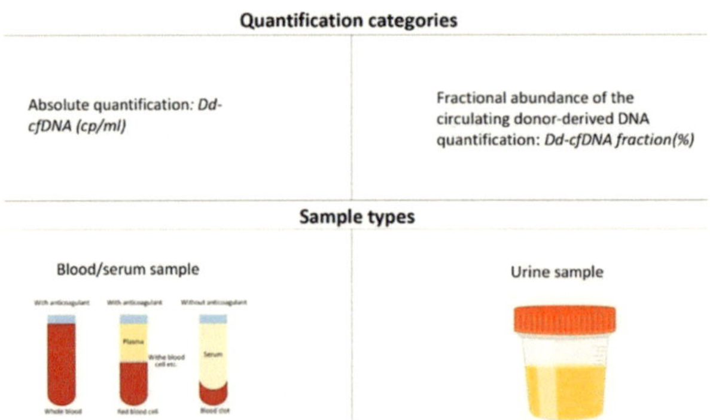

Figure 1.
Dd-cfDNA evaluation methods.

Particularly, for its detection in serum, various types of polymerase chain reaction (PCR) are available, and alternatively, an approach used for female recipients with male donors is the amplification of Y-chromosome specific genes [48]. Distinguishing the donor-derived cfDNA from the recipient-derived type is a process including the following steps. Firstly, SNP (single-nucleotide polymorphism) selection is conducted, followed by the targeted amplification and sequencing of the cfDNA samples [49]. The next step is the statistical determination of the recipient's heterozygous cutoff, on whose basis dd-cfDNA is estimated. Additionally, the value of the technique is increased by sample quality control and analytical validation [50]. Dd-cfDNA is a biomarker with a short half-life (<1.5 h), a characteristic adding accuracy in its clinical value [51]. Evaluation techniques of dd-cfDNA can be found in **Figure 1**.

8. Applications of dd-cfDNA evaluation in liver transplantation

Dd-cfDNA has many applications in the diagnosis of LT complications and in the monitoring of LT recipients. Those include early detection of pathological lesions, diagnosis of infections related to transplantation, monitoring of the patients, and cancer recurrence in cases of LT performed as treatment for hepatocellular cancer. **Figure 2** includes a scheme about applications of dd-cfDNA in LT.

8.1 Dd-cfDNA and subclinical graft injury evaluation

Subclinical graft injury refers to notable histological inflammation, while liver enzyme levels remain relatively normal, particularly under 2× ULN [52]. Using svLBxs, it has been observed that over 25% of liver transplant recipients with regular liver enzymes show graft injuries indicative of T-cell-mediated rejection (TCMR) [53, 54]. While svLBxs are very specific when it comes to detecting subclinical T-cell-mediated rejection (SubTCMR), their invasive nature and potential risks limit their frequent application in clinical settings. Dd-cfDNA emerges as a promising noninvasive marker for early identification of sub-TCMR. Several studies highlight a relationship between increased dd-cfDNA levels and sub-TCMR. For instance, there has been mentioned notably elevated fractional dd-cfDNA in patients exhibiting sub-TCMR, with a sensitivity and specificity of this method being 73 and 52%.

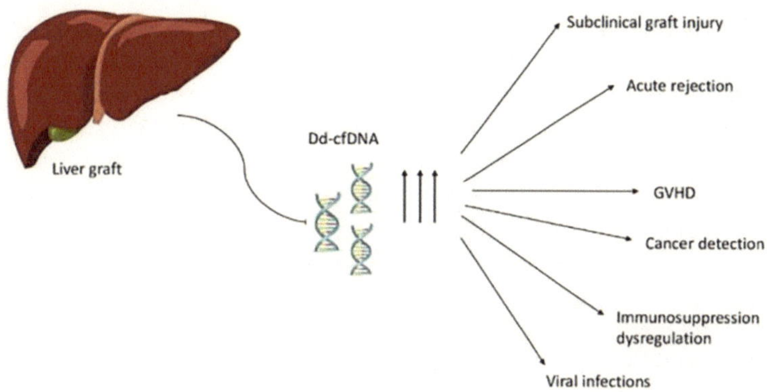

Figure 2.
Applications of dd-cfDNA in liver transplantation.

Despite the differences in fractional dd-cfDNA levels, there were no significant differences in absolute dd-cfDNA levels between those with or without graft damage [50]. Furthermore, during the investigation of personalized immunosuppressive treatment schemes, elevated graft cell-free DNA (GcfDNA) has been identified in cases of subclinical graft damage due to inadequate tacrolimus levels and connections between dd-cfDNA levels, tacrolimus concentrations, and the frequency of graft injuries have been also found, resulting in an optimal level of tacrolimus at around 6.8 μg/L [54, 55]. Moreover, increased GcfDNA percentage (graft cfDNA/total cfDNA) has been correlated with graft injury, reaching levels even above 50% after ischemia-reperfusion [54]. Lastly, short dd-cfDNA fractions specifically were also linked to graft impairments, indicating that small/large fragments ratio lower than 0.6 is correlated with stability of the graft function. [47].

8.2 Dd-cfDNA and diagnosis of rejection

In cases of rejection, and particularly acute rejection, the use of dd-cfDNA proved to be more sensitive and diagnostically valuable than liver function tests (LFTs), enabling an earlier and more accurate detection. Many studies have indicated that LT recipients experiencing acute rejection exhibit higher serum levels of dd-cfDNA compared to those without rejection, with the median dd-cfDNA percentage being three-fold higher comparing to before rejection diagnosis levels [50, 56–59]. The sensitivity and specificity of dd-cfDNA-based acute rejection diagnosis differentiated, ranging between 72 and 100% and 53–91% based on different cutoff levels. Additionally, it has been highlighted that dd-cfDNA serves not just as a non-invasive diagnostic tool for acute rejection but also allows for earlier detection than biopsies and conventional LFTs, detecting possible graft damage 1–2 days earlier than conventional methods [54]. A strategy to pinpoint the source of dd-cfDNA and diagnose complications in the recipient involves analyzing the fractions ratio, particularly patients undergoing acute rejection tend to have an elevated ratio of short fragments compared to individuals with healthy grafts [43].

8.3 Dd-cfDNA in graft versus host disease diagnosis

Graft versus host disease (GVHD) is a rare but life-threatening complication related to transplantation of mostly bone marrow and in rare cases solid organs [60]. It is recognized to have an asymptomatic phase, allowing for early identification and intervention by adjusting immunosuppressive drug levels [61]. Traditional methods for early GVHD detection, which rely on molecular techniques targeting macro chimerism, have been neither cost-effective nor feasible for routine clinical use [62]. Dd-cfDNA has been the center of a newly introduced, innovative diagnostic approach for GVHD detection. This method identifies GVHD based on criteria like increased serum dd-cfDNA levels, elevated proportions of donor-origin T and B cells, and the presence of donor-derived genomic-DNA (dd-gDNA) in skin samples. Such findings suggest the presence of multisystemic GVHD and potential concurrent infections. These strategies could serve as non-invasive tools for immune surveillance, facilitating quicker GVHD identification and thus resulting in an earlier treatment [48].

8.4 Dd-cfDNA in liver graft viral infections diagnosis

Transplant patients are following a medication scheme of continuous immunosuppression making them particularly susceptible to various opportunistic infections, including EBV and CMV. This susceptibility highlights the importance of having a non-invasive marker to assess potential viral infections in LT patients. There has been found that individuals with EBV or CMV exhibited notably elevated percentages and median quantities of dd-cfDNA, with CMV patients showing even higher levels than those with EBV (0.866 vs. 0.764 dd-cfDNA (cp/mL)) [63]. Furthermore, LT patients are prone to HCV infection. HCV-positive patients displayed a somewhat elevated and more variable GcfDNA proportion compared to those in stable health [54, 62].

8.5 Dd-cfDNA and early detection of cancer recurrence

It is known that liver transplantation is an evidence-based worldwide accepted treatment option for patients with liver tumors [64]. Usually, LT is performed in patients with hepatocellular cancer (HCC) according to Milan criteria, but in recent years, it has been applied in a series of patients with cholangiocarcinoma as well [65–67]. LT recipients require immunosuppression treatment in order to avoid rejection-related complications; thus, they are susceptible to cancer recurrence, with tumor recurrence rate after LT is estimated to be 8–20% [20, 21]. The gold standard of screening tests in these patients include imaging methods, tissue biopsies, and serum alpha-fetoprotein (AFP) follow-up [68]. Although those tests show great sensitivity and specificity in cancer detection, they result in radiation intake and many complications related to invasive biopsy procedure. Cell-free DNA (CfDNA), also referred to as liquid biopsy, appears to be an emerging biomarker of early, non-invasive diagnosis of cancer recurrence in LT recipients. Diagnostic approach of cancer is based on qualitative, with methylation profiles and different gene mutations being the main focus, and quantitative assessment, [69, 70]. CfDNA and other nucleic acid biomarkers diagnostic accuracy in HCC detection has been a field of research in the part, with promising results [70–75]. Apart from the diagnosis of cancer, those biomarkers have been used for the evaluation of biological activity and metastatic profile of the tumor [73]. When it comes to LT recipients, cfDNA-based diagnosis of cancer recurrence follows the same principles, with practically the tumor-related cfDNA being actually graft derived dd-cfDNA [64, 76–78]. Particularly, positive preoperative cfDNA is related to tumor characteristics such as larger size, multiple lesions, microvascular invasion, and advanced stages. Additionally, cfDNA is also a predictive factor for disease free and overall survival, with positive preoperative cfDNA status being correlated with shorter overall (mean 22.5 vs. 40.0 months) and disease-free survival (mean 16.6 vs. 35.3) [78].

8.6 Monitoring of immunosuppressant LT recipients

The value of evaluating dd-cfDNA clinically stems from its non-invasive nature and swift assessment. These attributes advocate for the inclusion of dd-cfDNA in routine monitoring for all LT recipients. Specifically, there has already been mentioned previously the significance of correlating dd-cfDNA concentrations with tacrolimus levels [79, 80]. Moreover, dd-cfDNA has been used for the personalization of dosage and monitoring of patients receiving tocilizumab and belatacept in kidney transplant recipients, with possible application to liver transplant recipients as well. [81, 82]. The success of tocilizumab treatment is evaluated with the decrease of levels of dd-cfDNA (%), with a decrease of 47% being reported after 12 months of treatment [81]. Although there are no specific official guidelines about the testing times for dd-cfDNA evaluation, days 7 and 14 after transplantation, followed by monthly testing over 6 months and every 3-month time points have been suggested [80].

9. Limitations of cfDNA application in everyday clinical practice

Even though dd-cfDNA can potentially be the gold standard in LT recipients monitoring, its application does not come without certain limitations. Firstly, due to factors like immunosuppression or underlying medical conditions, LT recipients may experience conditions such as leukopenia, leukocytosis, and inflammatory diseases, which could impact the accurate measurement of fractional dd-cfDNA. Additionally, as previously mentioned, while dd-cfDNA serves as a potential marker for various LT complications linked to graft damage, resulting in lack of specificity [83]. Moreover, there are specific scenarios in LT where dd-cfDNA might not serve as a viable biomarker, such as cases involving identical twin donors or donors and recipients from closely related families. Additionally, the use of dd-cfDNA for diagnosis becomes challenging in scenarios like dual organ transplants from a single donor or multiple organ transplants from diverse donors [84]. Lastly, dd-cfDNA is influenced by parameters like the size of the graft and its origin [55]. Higher peaks of dd-cfDNA in cases of deceased donor LT are most likely explained by higher levels of ischemia–reperfusion injury, but also by the fact that elevations in dd-cfDNA are more dramatic in larger grafts from deceased donors than from partial grafts in living donors [62, 85].

10. Conclusion

Although major progress has been made in the recent years when it comes to biomarkers research and particularly dd-cfDNA use in non-invasive monitoring of LT recipients, certain areas remain unexplored. The predominant focus of research lies on the use of dd-cfDNA for post-transplantation diagnosis. With the increase of the usage of machine perfusion, even in liver transplantation, dd-cfDNA could possibly serve as an useful biomarker for early pre-transplantation evaluation of the quality of the graft [86].

Another obstacle when it comes to clinical application of dd-cfDNA is the difficulty, expense, and time-intensive nature of its evaluation technique. Newly developed assays based on spectrophotometry, electrophoresis, or quantitative PCR (qPCR), next-generation sequencing, BEAMing (beads, emulsion, amplification, and magnetics), or droplet digital PCR (ddPCR), could possibly be applied in the dd-cfDNA assessment process and lead to faster accurate results [87, 88].

Lastly, the role of Artificial Intelligence (AI) in transplantation research is fundamental. AI has the potential to contribute significantly to the development of new applications of dd-cfDNA, with the formations of algorithms for graft evaluation based on dd-cfDNA values and with the detection of new genes and methylation patterns for the precise diagnosis of graft pathologies.

Conflict of interest

The authors declare no conflict of interest.

Author details

Eleni Avramidou*, Stella Vasileiadou and Georgios Tsoulfas
Department of Transplant Surgery, Center for Research and Innovation in Solid Organ Transplantation Aristotle University of Thessaloniki School of Medicine, Thessaloniki, Greece

*Address all correspondence to: avramidoue@auth.gr

References

[1] Starlz TE, Marchioro TL, Vonkaulla KN, Hermann G, Brittain RS, Wadell WR. Homotransplantation of the liver in humans. Surgery, Gynecology & Obstetrics. 1963;**117**:659-676

[2] Calne RY, Rolles K, White DJ, et al. Cyclosporin a initially as the only immunosuppressant in 34 recipients of cadaveric organs: 32 kidneys, 2 pancreases, and 2 livers. Lancet. 1979;**2**(8151):1033-1036. DOI: 10.1016/s0140-6736(79)92440-1

[3] International report on organ donation and Available at: https://www.transplant-observatory.org/wp-content/uploads/2022/12/2021-data-global-report-1.pdf [Accessed: 26 January 2024]

[4] Carotti S, Morini S, Carpino G, Gaudio E. Liver histology. In: Radu-Ionita F, Pyrsopoulos N, Jinga M, Tintoiu I, Sun Z, Bontas E, editors. Liver Diseases. Cham: Springer; 2020. DOI: 10.1007/978-3-030-24432-3_2

[5] Francis K. The anatomy and physiology of the liver. Philosophical Transactions of the Royal Society. 1833;**123**:123711-123770. DOI: 10.1098/rstl.1833.0031

[6] Mall FP. A study of the structural unit of the liver. American Journal of Anatomy. 1906;**5**:227-308

[7] Poisson J et al. Liver sinusoidal endothelial cells: Physiology and role in liver diseases. Journal of Hepatology. 2017;**66**(1):212-227. DOI: 10.1016/j.jhep.2016.07.009

[8] Dixon LJ, Barnes M, Tang H, Pritchard MT, Nagy LE. Kupffer cells in the liver. Comprehensive Physiology. 2013;**3**(2):785-797. DOI: 10.1002/cphy.c120026

[9] Peng H, Wisse E, Tian Z. Liver natural killer cells: Subsets and roles in liver immunity. Cellular & Molecular Immunology. 2016;**13**:328-336. DOI: 10.1038/cmi.2015.96

[10] Alvaro D, Mancino MG, Glaser S, et al. Proliferating cholangiocytes: A neuroendocrine compartment in the diseased liver. Gastroenterology. 2007;**132**(1):415-431. DOI: 10.1053/j.gastro.2006.07.023

[11] Kupiec-Weglinski JW, Busuttil RW. Ischemia and reperfusion injury in liver transplantation. Transplantation Proceedings. 2005;**37**(4):1653-1656. DOI: 10.1016/j.transproceed.2005.03.134

[12] Kageyama S, Kadono K, Hirao H, et al. Ischemia-reperfusion injury in allogeneic liver transplantation: A role of CD4 T cells in early allograft injury. Transplantation. 2021;**105**(9):1989-1997. DOI: 10.1097/TP.0000000000003488

[13] Abu-Amara M, Yang SY, Tapuria N, Fuller B, Davidson B, Seifalian A. Liver ischemia/reperfusion injury: Processes in inflammatory networks--a review. Liver Transplantation. 2010;**16**(9):1016-1032. DOI: 10.1002/lt.22117

[14] Shetty S, Adams DH, Hubscher SG. Post-transplant liver biopsy and the immune response: Lessons for the clinician. Expert Review of Clinical Immunology. 2012;**8**(7):645-661. DOI: 10.1586/eci.12.65

[15] Heidt S, Hester J, Shankar S, Friend PJ, Wood KJ. B cell repopulation after alemtuzumab induction-transient increase in transitional B cells and long-term dominance of naïve B cells. American Journal of

Transplantation. 2012;**12**(7):1784-1792. DOI: 10.1111/j.1600-6143.2012.04012.x

[16] O'Leary JG, Kaneku H, Demetris AJ, et al. Antibody-mediated rejection as a contributor to previously unexplained early liver allograft loss. Liver Transplantation. 2014;**20**(2):218-227. DOI: 10.1002/lt.23788

[17] Onpoaree N, Sanpavat A, Sintusek P. Cytomegalovirus infection in liver-transplanted children. World Journal of Hepatology. 2022;**14**(2):338-353. DOI: 10.4254/wjh.v14.i2.338

[18] Berumen J, Baglieri J, Kisseleva T, Mekeel K. Liver fibrosis: Pathophysiology and clinical implications. WIREs Mechanisms of Disease. 2021;**13**:e1499. DOI: 10.1002/wsbm.1499

[19] Irshad M, Gupta P, Irshad K. Immunopathogenesis of liver injury during hepatitis C virus infection. Viral Immunology. 2019;**32**(3):112-120. DOI: 10.1089/vim.2018.0124

[20] Sapisochin G, Goldaracena N, Laurence JM, et al. The extended Toronto criteria for liver transplantation in patients with hepatocellular carcinoma: A prospective validation study. Hepatology. 2016;**64**(6):2077-2088. DOI: 10.1002/hep.28643

[21] Silva MF, Sherman M. Criteria for liver transplantation for HCC: What should the limits be? Journal of Hepatology. 2011;**55**(5):1137-1147. DOI: 10.1016/j.jhep.2011.05.012

[22] Calderaro J et al. Molecular and histological correlations in liver cancer. Journal of Hepatology. 2019;**71**(3):616-630. DOI: 10.1016/j.jhep.2019.06.001

[23] Pratt DS, Kaplan MM. Evaluation of abnormal liver-enzyme results in asymptomatic patients. The New England Journal of Medicine. 2000;**342**(17):1266-1271. DOI: 10.1056/NEJM200004273421707

[24] Center SA. Interpretation of liver enzymes. Veterinary Clinics of North America: Small Animal Practice. 2007b;**37**(2):297-333. DOI: 10.1016/j.cvsm.2006.11.009

[25] Rocque B, Zaldana A, Weaver C, et al. Clinical value of surveillance biopsies in Pediatric liver transplantation. Liver Transplantation. 2022;**28**(5):843-854. DOI: 10.1002/lt.26399

[26] Gracia-Sancho J, Casillas-Ramírez A, Peralta C. Molecular pathways in protecting the liver from ischaemia/reperfusion injury: A 2015 update. Clinical Science (London, England). 2015;**129**(4):345-362. DOI: 10.1042/CS20150223

[27] de Miranda FS, Barauna VG, dos Santos L, Costa G, Vassallo PF, Campos LCG. Properties and application of cell-free DNA as a clinical biomarker. International Journal of Molecular Sciences. 2021;**22**(17):9110. DOI: 10.3390/ijms22179110

[28] Aronson JK, Ferner RE. Biomarkers—A general review. Current Protocols in Pharmacology. 2017;**76**(1):9.23.1-9.23.17. DOI: 10.1002/cpph.19

[29] Lin Z, Li H, He C, et al. Metabolomic biomarkers for the diagnosis and post-transplant outcomes of AFP negative hepatocellular carcinoma. Front. Oncologia. 2023;**13**:1072775. Published 2023 Feb 9. DOI: 10.3389/fonc.2023.1072775

[30] Zhu H, Wang M, Xiong X, et al. Plasma metabolomic profiling reveals factors associated with dose-adjusted trough concentration of tacrolimus in

liver transplant recipients. Frontiers in Pharmacology. 2022;**13**:1045843. Published 2022 Oct 31. DOI: 10.3389/fphar.2022.1045843

[31] De Stefano N, Calleri A, Faini AC, et al. Extracellular vesicles in liver transplantation: Current evidence and future challenges. International Journal of Molecular Sciences. 2023;**24**(17):13547. Published 2023 August 31. DOI: 10.3390/ijms241713547

[32] Budkowska M, Ostrycharz E, Serwin NM, et al. Biomarkers of the complement system activation (C3a, C5a, sC5b-9) in serum of patients before and after liver transplantation. Biomedicine. 2023;**11**(7):2070. Published 2023 July 23. DOI: 10.3390/biomedicines11072070

[33] Yu J, Shi X, Ma J, et al. C-reactive protein is an independent predictor of 30-day bacterial infection post-liver transplantation. Biomolecules. 2021;**11**(8):1195. Published 2021 Aug 12. DOI: 10.3390/biom11081195

[34] Boix F, Legaz I, Minhas A, et al. Identification of peripheral CD154+ T cells and HLA-DRB1 as biomarkers of acute cellular rejection in adult liver transplant recipients. Clinical and Experimental Immunology. 2021;**203**(2):315-328. DOI: 10.1111/cei.13533

[35] Decker SO, Krüger A, Wilk H, et al. Concurrent change in serum cholinesterase activity and Midregional-Proadrennomedullin level could predict patient outcome following liver transplantation. Biomolecules. 2022;**12**(7):989. Published 2022 Jul 15. DOI: 10.3390/biom12070989

[36] Wang W, Wang B, Liu C, et al. Serum proteomic predicts effectiveness and reveals potential biomarkers for complications in liver transplant patients. Aging (Albany NY). 2020;**12**(12):12119-12141. DOI: 10.18632/aging.103381

[37] Morsiani C, Collura S, Sevini F, et al. Circulating miR-122-5p, miR-92a-3p, and miR-18a-5p as potential biomarkers in human liver transplantation follow-up. International Journal of Molecular Sciences. 2023;**24**(4):3457. Published 2023 Feb 9. DOI: 10.3390/ijms24043457

[38] Keshavarz Z, Zareei N, Afshari A, Karimi MH, Yaghobi R, Malekhosseini SA. TLR2 and TLR4 mRNA expression levels in liver transplant patients with acute rejection. Immunobiology. 2021;**226**(4):152107. DOI: 10.1016/j.imbio.2021.152107

[39] McClure T, Goh SK, Cox D, Muralidharan V, Dobrovic A, Testro AG. Donor-specific cell-free DNA as a biomarker in liver transplantation: A review. World Journal of Transplantation. 2020;**10**(11):307-319. DOI: 10.5500/wjt.v10.i11.307

[40] Huang A, Guo DZ, Zhang X, et al. Serial circulating tumor DNA profiling predicts tumor recurrence after liver transplantation for liver cancer. Hepatology International. Published online November; 2023;**18**:254-264. DOI: 10.1007/s12072-023-10594-x

[41] Wehrle CJ, Raj R, Aykun N, et al. Liquid biopsy by ctDNA in liver transplantation for colorectal cancer liver metastasis. Journal of Gastrointestinal Surgery. 2023;**27**(7):1498-1509. DOI: 10.1007/s11605-023-05723-8

[42] Avramidou E, Vasileiadou S, Antoniadis N, Katsanos G, Kofinas A, Karakasi K-E, et al. Liver transplantation and dd-cfDNA: A small solution for a big problem. Liver. 2023;**3**(1):76-81. DOI: 10.3390/livers3010007

[43] Fernández-Galán E, Badenas C, Fondevila C, Jiménez W, Navasa M,

Puig-Butillé JA, et al. Monitoring of donor-derived cell-free DNA by short tandem repeats: Concentration of Total cell-free DNA and fragment size for acute rejection risk assessment in liver transplantation. Liver Transplantation. 2022;**28**(2):257-268. DOI: 10.1002/lt.26272

[44] Sigdel TK, Vitalone MJ, Tran TQ, et al. A rapid noninvasive assay for the detection of renal transplant injury. Transplantation. 2013;**96**(1):97-101. DOI: 10.1097/TP.0b013e318295ee5a

[45] Grskovic M, Hiller DJ, Eubank LA, et al. Validation of a clinical-grade assay to measure donor-derived cell-free DNA in solid organ transplant recipients. The Journal of Molecular Diagnostics. 2016;**18**(6):890-902. DOI: 10.1016/j.jmoldx.2016.07.003

[46] Kueng N, Arcioni S, Sandberg F, et al. Comparison of methods for donor-derived cell-free DNA quantification in plasma and urine from solid organ transplant recipients. Frontiers in Genetics. 2023;**14**:1089830. Published 2023 Jan 27. DOI: 10.3389/fgene.2023.1089830

[47] Ng HI et al. Analysis of fragment size distribution of cell-free DNA: A potential non-invasive marker to monitor graft damage in living-related liver transplantation for inborn errors of metabolism. Molecular Genetics and Metabolism. 2019;**127**(1):45-50. DOI: 10.1016/j.ymgme.2019.03.004

[48] Lewis D et al. High levels of donor-derived cell-free DNA in a case of graft-versus-host-disease following liver transplantation. American Journal of Transplantation. 2022b;**22**(3):973-976. DOI: 10.1111/ajt.16894

[49] Altuğ Y, Liang N, Ram R, et al. Analytical validation of a single-nucleotide polymorphism-based donor-derived cell-free DNA assay for detecting rejection in kidney transplant patients. Transplantation. 2019;**103**(12):2657-2665. DOI: 10.1097/TP.0000000000002665

[50] Baumann AK, Beck J, Kirchner T, Hartleben B, Schütz E, Oellerich M, et al. Elevated fractional donor-derived cell-free DNA during subclinical graft injury after liver transplantation. Liver Transplantation. 2022;**28**(12):1911-1919. DOI: 10.1002/lt.26479

[51] Lehmann-Werman R, Magenheim J, Moss J, et al. Monitoring liver damage using hepatocyte-specific methylation markers in cell-free circulating DNA. JCI. Insight. 2018;**3**(12):e120687. Published 2018 Jun 21. DOI: 10.1172/jci.insight.120687

[52] Londoño M-C et al. Molecular profiling of subclinical inflammatory lesions in long-term surviving adult liver transplant recipients. Journal of Hepatology. 2018;**69**(3):626-634. DOI: 10.1016/j.jhep.2018.04.012

[53] Saunders EA et al. Outcome and safety of a surveillance biopsy guided personalized immunosuppression program after liver transplantation. American Journal of Transplantation. 2022;**22**(2):519-531. DOI: 10.1111/ajt.16817

[54] Schütz E et al. Graft-derived cell-free DNA, a noninvasive early rejection and graft damage marker in liver transplantation: A prospective, observational, Multicenter cohort study. PLoS Medicine. 2017;**14**(4):e1002286. DOI: 10.1371/journal.pmed.1002286

[55] Oellerich M, Schütz E, Kanzow P, Schmitz J, Beck J, Kollmar O, et al. Use of graft-derived cell-free DNA as an organ integrity biomarker to

Reexamine effective tacrolimus trough concentrations after liver transplantation. Therapeutic Drug Monitoring. 2014;**36**(2):136-140. DOI: 10.1097/FTD.0000000000000044

[56] Höfer A, Jonigk D, Hartleben B, et al. Non-invasive screening for subclinical liver graft injury in adults via donor-specific anti-HLA antibodies. Scientific Reports. 2020;**10**:14242. DOI: 10.1038/s41598-020-70938-7

[57] Kanamori H, Yamada Y, Ito Y, et al. Noninvasive graft monitoring using donor-derived cell-free DNA in Japanese liver transplantation. Hepatology Research. 2024;**54**(3):300-314. DOI: 10.1111/hepr.13978

[58] Taylor AL, Gibbs P, Sudhindran S, Key T, Goodman RS, Morgan CH, et al. Monitoring systemic donor lymphocyte macrochimerism to aid the diagnosis of graftversus-host disease after liver transplantation. Transplantation. 2004;**77**(3):441-445. DOI: 10.1097/01.TP.0000103721.29729.FE

[59] Cox DRA, McClure T, Zhang F, et al. Graft-derived cell-free DNA quantification following liver transplantation using tissue-specific DNA methylation and donor-specific genotyping techniques: An orthogonal comparison study. Epigenomes. 2023;**7**(2):11. Published 2023 Jun 9. DOI: 10.3390/epigenomes7020011

[60] Hülsdünker J, Zeiser R. Insights into the pathogenesis of gvhd: What mice can teach us about man. Tissue Antigens. 2014;**85**(1):2-9. DOI: 10.1111/tan.12497

[61] Taylor AL, Gibbs P, Bradley JA. Acute graft versus host disease following liver transplantation: The enemy within. American Journal of Transplantation. 2004;**4**(4):466-474. DOI: 10.1111/j.1600-6143.2004.00406.x

[62] Oellerich M, Walson PD, Beck J, Schmitz J, Kollmar O, Schütz E. Graft-derived cell-free DNA as a marker of transplant graft injury. Therapeutic Drug Monitoring. 2016;**38** (Suppl. 1):S75-S79. DOI: 10.1097/FTD.0000000000000239

[63] Zhao D, Zhou T, Luo Y, et al. Preliminary clinical experience applying donor-derived cell-free DNA to discern rejection in pediatric liver transplant recipients. Scientific Reports. 2021;**11**:1138. DOI: 10.1038/s41598-020-80845-6

[64] Abdelrahim M, Esmail A, Abudayyeh A, et al. Transplant oncology: An emerging discipline of cancer treatment. Cancers (Basel). 2023;**15**(22):5337. Published 2023 Nov 9. DOI: 10.3390/cancers15225337

[65] Xu X, Lu D, Ling Q, et al. Liver transplantation for hepatocellular carcinoma beyond the Milan criteria. Gut. 2016;**65**(6):1035-1041. DOI: 10.1136/gutjnl-2014-308513

[66] Mazzaferro V, Regalia E, Doci R, et al. Liver transplantation for the treatment of small hepatocellular carcinomas in patients with cirrhosis. The New England Journal of Medicine. 1996;**334**(11):693-699. DOI: 10.1056/NEJM199603143341104

[67] Eletta OA, Panayotova GG, Lunsford KE. Liver transplant for intrahepatic Cholangiocarcinoma. The Surgical Clinics of North America. 2024;**104**(1):215-225. DOI: 10.1016/j.suc.2023.07.006

[68] Filgueira NA. Hepatocellular carcinoma recurrence after liver transplantation: Risk factors, screening and clinical presentation. World Journal of Hepatology. 2019;**11**(3):261-272. DOI: 10.4254/wjh.v11.i3.261

[69] Luo B, Ma F, Liu H, et al. Cell-free DNA methylation markers for differential diagnosis of hepatocellular carcinoma. BMC Medicine. 2022;**20**(1):8. Published 2022 Jan 14. DOI: 10.1186/s12916-021-02201-3

[70] Zhang X, Wang Z, Tang W, et al. Ultrasensitive and affordable assay for early detection of primary liver cancer using plasma cell-free DNA fragmentomics. Hepatology. 2022;**76**(2):317-329. DOI: 10.1002/hep.32308

[71] Ng CKY, Di Costanzo GG, Terracciano LM, Piscuoglio S. Circulating cell-free DNA in hepatocellular carcinoma: Current insights and outlook. Frontiers in Medicine (Lausanne). 2018;**5**:78. Published 2018 Mar 26. DOI: 10.3389/fmed.2018.00078

[72] Lu CY, Chen SY, Peng HL, Kan PY, Chang WC, Yen CJ. Cell-free methylation markers with diagnostic and prognostic potential in hepatocellular carcinoma. Oncotarget. 2017;**8**(4):6406-6418. DOI: 10.18632/oncotarget.14115

[73] Zhou C, Weng J, Liu S, et al. Whole-exome sequencing reveals the metastatic potential of hepatocellular carcinoma from the perspective of tumor and circulating tumor DNA. Hepatology International. 2023;**17**(6):1461-1476. DOI: 10.1007/s12072-023-10540-x

[74] Bae M, Kim G, Lee TR, et al. Integrative modeling of tumor genomes and epigenomes for enhanced cancer diagnosis by cell-free DNA. Nature Communications. 2023, 2017. Published 2023 Apr 10;**14**(1). Article number: 2017 (2023). DOI: 10.1038/s41467-023-37768-3

[75] Zhu GQ, Liu WR, Tang Z, et al. Serial circulating tumor DNA to predict early recurrence in patients with hepatocellular carcinoma: A prospective study. Molecular Oncology. 2022;**16**(2):549-561. DOI: 10.1002/1878-0261.13105

[76] Manzi J, Hoff CO, Ferreira R, et al. Cell-free DNA as a surveillance tool for hepatocellular carcinoma patients after liver transplant. Cancers (Basel). 2023;**15**(12):3165. Published 2023 Jun 13. DOI: 10.3390/cancers15123165

[77] Reddy T, Esmail A, Chang JC, Ghobrial RM, Abdelrahim M. Utility of cell-free DNA detection in transplant oncology. Cancers (Basel). 2022;**14**(3):743. DOI: 10.3390/cancers14030743

[78] Wang J, Huang A, Wang YP, et al. Circulating tumor DNA correlates with microvascular invasion and predicts tumor recurrence of hepatocellular carcinoma. Annals of Translational Medicine. 2020;**8**(5):237. DOI: 10.21037/atm.2019.12.154

[79] Oellerich M, Shipkova M, Asendorf T, et al. Absolute quantification of donor-derived cell-free DNA as a marker of rejection and graft injury in kidney transplantation: Results from a prospective observational study. American Journal of Transplantation. 2019;**19**(11):3087-3099. DOI: 10.1111/ajt.15416

[80] Oellerich M, Budde K, Osmanodja B, et al. Donor-derived cell-free DNA for personalized immunosuppression in renal transplantation. Therapeutic Drug Monitoring. 2023;**45**(1):20-25. DOI: 10.1097/FTD.0000000000001023

[81] Boonpheng B, De Castro ICC, Ng YH, et al. Tocilizumab for treatment of chronic active antibody-mediated rejection in kidney transplant

recipients. Clinical Transplantation. 2023;**37**(5):e14936. DOI: 10.1111/ctr.14936

[82] Osmanodja B et al. Donor-derived cell-free DNA for kidney allograft surveillance after conversion to belatacept: Prospective pilot study. Journal of Clinical Medicine. 2023;**12**(6):2437. DOI: 10.3390/jcm12062437

[83] Kanzow P, Kollmar O, Schütz E, Oellerich M, Schmitz J, Beck J, et al. Graft-derived cell-free DNA as an early organ integrity biomarker after transplantation of a marginal HELLP syndrome donor liver. Transplantation. 2014;**98**(5):e43-e45. DOI: 10.1097/TP.0000000000000303

[84] Oellerich M et al. Donor-derived cell-free DNA as a diagnostic tool in transplantation. Frontiers in Genetics. 2022;**13**:1031894. DOI: 10.3389/fgene.2022.1031894

[85] Ng H-I, Sun L-Y, Zhu Z-J. Detecting graft-derived cell-free DNA through amplification refractory mutation system polymerase chain reaction in living-donor liver transplantation: Report of 2 cases. Transplantation Proceedings. 2019;**51**(3):820-822. DOI: 10.1016/j.transproceed.2018.11.011

[86] Da Silva S, Richard X, Weber A, Dutkowski P, Clavien P-A. Machine perfusion in liver transplantation. Hepatology. 2022;**76**(5):1531-1549. DOI: 10.1002/hep.32546

[87] Mojtabanezhad Shariatpanahi A, Rokni P, Shahabi E, et al. Simple and cost-effective laboratory methods to evaluate and validate cell-free DNA isolation. BMC Research Notes. 2018;**11**:757. DOI: 10.1186/s13104-018-3866-8

[88] Mauger F et al. Comprehensive evaluation of methods to isolate, quantify, and characterize circulating cell-free DNA from small volumes of plasma. Analytical and Bioanalytical Chemistry. 2015;**407**(22):6873-6878. DOI: 10.1007/s00216-015-8846-4

Chapter 5

Emergencies Following Orthotopic Liver Transplant

Brian L. Shaw, Bill S. Majdalany and Carlos E. Marroquin

Abstract

Complications following lifesaving liver transplantation can be devastating and must be managed properly to optimize the patient and allograft survival. There are non-immune, non-infectious complications which present a severe risk to survival of both the patient and the allograft. These include primary graft non-function (PNF) and hepatic artery thrombosis (HAT). Other complications manifest less urgently but continue to represent potentially lethal consequences to both the patient and the hepatic allograft. These include vena cava outflow disruptions, portal venous outflow derangements, and portal vein thrombosis (PVT). Successful management of these complications is optimized with a multidisciplinary approach to the care of liver transplant recipients. We describe their definition, epidemiology, pathophysiology, related factors, presentation, operative and non-operative management, outcomes, and future directions of these potentially catastrophic complications.

Keywords: re transplant, hepatic artery thrombisis, primary non function, portal vein thrombosis, vena cava outflow disruptions, portal venous outflow derangements

1. Introduction

Medical management of patients with end stage liver diseases has improved allowing more patients to survive to a point where a liver transplant has become the next expected treatment. We are embarking on an era that is experiencing better medical and multimodal management of patients with metastatic malignancies to the liver with no extrahepatic disease. As such, more patients are waiting on the wait list for a liver transplant motivating transplant centers to push the boundaries and utilize what were once marginal organs for transplantation. Technological advances in the field of machine perfusion and normothermic regional organ recovery will increase the utilization of donors after cardiac death. Moreover, centers are innovating with the use of living donors and cadaveric donors that were once thought to be suboptimal donors to transplant patients once thought to be prohibitive transplant candidates. This has led to new collaborations across all medical fields including Interventional Radiology and has resulted in the creation of new subdisciplines such as Transplant Oncology. With these efforts, we will invariably experience complications that will mandate an equally robust comprehensive collaboration to obtain the best possible outcomes.

 IntechOpen

1.1 Primary graft nonfunction (PNF)

Given the promise of a new beginning that liver transplantation offers, it is devastating when liver transplants never function. The evolution of primary nonfunction is complicated as the etiologies are compounded in nature and origin. The syndrome of graft dysfunction resides on a spectrum from early allograft dysfunction (EAD) to the most severe form, primary graft nonfunction (PNF) that occurs in the immediate perioperative period following reperfusion of the transplanted liver and represents a surgical emergency [1]. The incidence of PNF has declined over the years but the impact on patients and the limited organ pool remains substantial.

According to the definition from Ploeg et al. [2] PNF is diagnosed in liver allografts that fail to sustain their function, leading to death or re-transplantation within 7 days of the primary operation. The classification has been variably defined as others allow for 10, 14, or even 30 days from primary operation for allograft dysfunction leading to graft failure to define PNF [3–6]. The clinical and time parameters to diagnose PNF remain variable and are characterized differently throughout the world and represent an area for greater consensus. In the United Kingdom, a study of 1286 primary liver transplants developed a statistical model using transplant albumin, day-1 aspartate aminotransferase (AST), day-1 lactate, day-3 bilirubin, day-3 international normalized ratio (INR), and day-7 AST that achieved improved sensitivity (73%) compared to the existing UK (31%) and US (66%) diagnostic criteria without reduction in specificity (95% compared to UK 93% and US 98%) [7]. The histologic findings from biopsies and assessment of explanted livers corroborate the clinical endpoint, a lack of function, with necrosis in the absence of vascular complications, cholestasis, inflammatory infiltrates, and even microvascular steatosis [8, 9]. The syndrome of PNF is multifactorial in origin and requires multidisciplinary efforts to assess, predict, and treat this complex pathology.

The etiology of PNF is not entirely clear and while it is likely multifactorial in nature, ischemia-reperfusion injury (IRI) is a leading culprit in the etiology of PNF. IRI is defined as a reoxygenation injury where tissue damage occurs upon re-establishing blood supply following a period of absent blood flow during post recovery cold storage. Hepatocytes and liver sinusoidal endothelial cells (LSECs) are significantly damaged during IRI. Hepatocytes have been shown to be more susceptible to warm ischemic damage and LSECs more prone to cold ischemic damage [10]. Livers sustain a period of hypoxia during the recovery and preservation process. This lack of oxygen prevents oxidative phosphorylation and results in ATP depletion, anaerobic metabolism, and alterations in electrolyte homeostasis [11]. These changes result in cellular swelling and impaired function. During implantation of the allograft reperfusion injury is also mediated by reactive oxygen species (ROS) that damage cells, release proinflammatory mediators, cause microcirculatory dysfunction, and result in cell death [11]. A study by Ali et al. [12] correlated the severity of IRI in time-zero liver transplants and found the presence of severe IRI was statistically significant for the occurrence of PNF and need for 90-day re-transplantation. That study defined IRI as a global assessment of the histopathologic presence of neutrophilic infiltrate, apoptosis, and hepatocyte cell dropout. Similarly, Ito et al. [13] defined IRI by infiltration of inflammatory cells including neutrophils, monocytes, and T cells, with early damage to Kupffer cells and sinusoidal epithelial cells. They confirmed the presence of moderate/severe IRI in 42.9% of patients with primary allograft dysfunction compared to 24.8% in those with only minor IRI.

As the pathophysiology of PNF continues to undergo evaluation, much of the study on this topic aims to describe related factors. Reperfusion injury, cold/warm ischemia times, donor age, hepatic steatosis, serum sodium levels, recipient nutritional status, and many more have been associated with PNF in the literature. The Donor Risk Index (DRI) was introduced by Feng et al. [14] in 2006 to predict the risk of graft failure and is based on a scored system of donor related factors. The DRI provides solid quantitative prognostic information for allograft allocation.

However, the donor risk index is estimated for the average waiting candidate and does not appropriately capture many unique elements of the donor and recipient risk profile, such as older age donors and donors with hepatitis, representing a continued challenge in assessing and preventing PNF [15]. Furthermore, the quality of a graft and its recipient is a complex topic that relies on clinical experience to evaluate a recipient's reserve and ability to tolerate the metabolic and inflammatory insults that may occur with varying quality allografts. Additional algorithms to assist in matching donor and recipient characteristics have been developed for this reason but the process remains an imperfect science [16].

Cold ischemic times (CIT) and warm ischemic times (WIT) have been found to affect EAD and PNF. CIT is defined by the absence of blood flow while the organ is in cold storage until reperfusion and begins at the time of cross clamping during the donor recovery. WIT begins at the time the organ is removed from cold storage and ends with the initiation of graft reperfusion. Ischemic insults to a donor organ involve controllable and uncontrollable parameters. Both cold and warm ischemia times can be modified to a certain degree with improved processes and highly skilled teams. Two studies by Bastos-Neves et al. [17] and Sirivatanauksorn et al. [18] did show differences in allograft dysfunction with warm ischemia times >40 minutes and > 45 minutes respectively. Most of the literature agrees that the total warm ischemic time should be <60 minutes [19]. In comparison, the total cold ischemic time is more variable in the literature based on donor type. Overall, cold ischemia times >10 hours have been shown to be associated with increased rates of PNF [3, 20]. Johnson et al. [4] found a significant difference in PNF occurrence with cold ischemic times of 8.40 ± 0.14 hrs compared to 7.71 ± 0.03 hrs ($P = 0.0001$). In donors after cardiac death (DCD) or non-heart beating donors, cold ischemic time aims are shorter (<6 hours compared <8 or 12 hours) as these grafts do not tolerate the same duration of cold ischemia that non-cardiac death allografts allow [21].

Increasing donor age has been widely discussed as a risk factor for graft dysfunction. Aging is associated with hepatocyte senescence and diminished regeneration, making older age a susceptible factor to the consequences of organ donation. Donor age has been shown to negatively impact outcomes in liver transplants over the entire age range in multiple large studies and is a component of the DRI [14, 22, 23]. In an analysis of over 11,000 liver transplants utilizing the Scientific Registry of Transplant Recipients (SRTR), donor age > 40 years was a strong predictor of graft loss and death in individuals transplanted for liver failure secondary to viral hepatitis [24]. Additionally, in a national review of 5150 liver transplants performed in Spain, donor age > 50 years and > 70 years was associated with an increasing risk of graft loss (RR = 1.27 and 1.4, respectively) [25]. However, with advances in modern medicine and populations living healthier, longer lives, what constitutes an older donor is unclear. Additionally, studies on donor age and graft loss in liver transplantation have seldomly studied PNF as an etiology. In a recent study by Houben et al. [26] the authors stratified liver transplant donors into two groups, (65–69 years and ≥ 70 years) and found no statistical difference for rates of PNF between the groups. Additionally, that study found that one-year patient survival was not statistically different for donors <65 years and donors of 65–69 years (77.1% vs. 78.5%).

Furthermore, multiple other studies have shown a lack of association with donor age and an increased incidence in PNF [25, 27–29]. Yet, older age remains a risk factor for the complications of organ transplantation but remains a monumental challenge to weigh against the high demand for organs as the discrepancy between organ supply and demand continues to grow.

The effects of hepatic steatosis on overall hepatic health and function are well documented. Obesity induced uncoupling protein-2 (UCP2) mRNA and protein expression causes inefficient consumption of high energy phosphates leading to steatosis. This mechanism is exacerbated during organ preservation, ischemia, and reperfusion that has shown an increased incidence in PNF from transplanted fatty livers [30]. Past literature has documented increased rates of PNF with worsening percentages of hepatic steatosis taken from graft biopsies prior to transplantation [2, 31]. Generally, macrosteatosis up to 30% is considered safe for transplantation, whereas >30% and > 60% incrementally increase the risk for graft failure, respectively [32]. However, due to a growing organ shortage, the use of organs for transplantation has become more liberal in recent years and the acceptability of steatotic grafts has varied. A recent study by Kulik et al. [33] showed even minor graft macrosteatosis to be significantly associated with PNF. Additionally, microsteaosis has also been shown to increase the risk of early allograft dysfunction after transplantation [34]. Yet, in the study by Westerkamp et al. [35] comparison of grafts with moderate steatosis (30–60% macrosteatosis) to grafts without any signs of steatosis revealed no increase in the occurrence of PNF (5% vs. 5%). Finally, a study by McCormack et al. [36] found that transplanted livers with severe steatosis (> 60%) that would have been discarded by most transplant centers provided comparable sixty-day and 3-year survivals with recipients of non-steatotic grafts. However, while a percentage of these allografts functioned providing reasonable survivals, this cohort also had significantly higher rates of primary graft dysfunction including rates of PNF. Although hepatic steatosis is undoubtably a risk factor for the development of graft dysfunction, the evaluation is somewhat individually dependent, and the interplay by effecting ischemic times exists, thus entirely relying on the degree of steatosis for transplant is unclear. Additionally, recipients with better condition and reserve, may be able to endure lesser quality grafts with higher steatosis while they recover during the immediate post-transplant period, again leading to an imperfect allocation process that still requires experienced transplant clinician decision making.

Donor serum sodium levels have also been associated with postoperative graft dysfunction. Hypernatremia at the time of organ recovery is associated with poor outcomes and is additionally included in the DRI proposed by Feng et al. [14, 37] However, studies have also shown that correcting the sodium level prior to explanting the donor liver results in no increase in allograft dysfunction and no decrease in patient survival [38].

In 2002, the MELD score was adopted by UNOS to quantify the severity of liver disease and drive allocation. Olthoff et al. [39] found that the recipient MELD score is also associated with the evolution of EAD, demonstrating that it is not just donor characteristics, but also the status of the recipient that contributes to graft dysfunction following transplantation. The incidence of PNF after primary liver transplantation continues to vary in the literature, but most recent studies show an incidence of 3.5% – 9.1% of all primary liver transplantations [3, 4, 6, 7, 14]. Many recipient factors have been implicated in the occurrence of PNF. In a paper by Markmann et al. [40] primary graft survival was reduced by the combination of recipient creatinine greater than 2.0 mg/dL and pretransplant mechanical ventilation. In a review of transplantation for fulminant hepatic failure, 13.2% of grafts were lost to PNF, and the analysis found ethnicity/race, time from jaundice to encephalopathy, intracranial pressure (ICP) monitoring, veno-veno bypass (VVBP), and donor age were found to have significant influence on graft survival [41].

Nutritional status is a well-known component of overall health, especially within the realm of surgical outcomes. In fact, the European Society for Parenteral and Enteral Nutrition (ESPEN) has guidelines for organ transplantation recommend nutritional supplementation to improve nutritional status and liver function in recipients [42]. Experimental studies have also demonstrated beneficial effects of vitamins C and E supplementation. Interestingly, protein restricted diets may be protective and mitigate against hepatic ischemia and reperfusion injury which are the underpinnings of PNF [43, 44]. Thus, poor nutritional optimization leading up to transplantation increases the risk of hepatic injury and possibly PNF due to ischemic, reperfusion injury [45]. However, other studies are contradictory, showing exacerbations in ischemia and reperfusion injury to the liver with appropriate and varying diets perioperatively [46]. Thus, specific diets in the liver transplant recipient are still a matter of debate. Study of the gut microbiome is an emerging field and one that may unlock future insights to transplant related complications. Studies have shown the gut microbiota may contribute to the generation of memory alloreactive T cells that have been implicated in transplant rejection, and that the intestinal microbiome is altered after allogenic transplantation [47]. How nutrition and the gut microbiome is related to PNF is still unknown but represents an area for future research.

Additionally, functional capacity/status and rehabilitation are known factors in surgical outcomes and are especially important for the massive metabolic stress that comes with solid organ transplantation. In a study by Jacob et al. [48] Posttransplant mortality increased from 5.3% in patients able to carry out normal activity without restriction to 24.8% in patients completely reliant on nursing and medical care. Thus, emphasizing pre- and postoperative functional capacity along with nutritional optimization are additional parameters to improve overall outcomes in liver transplantation.

Regardless of the inciting factors, the mainstay of management of PNF relies on identifying allograft dysfunction early, beginning aggressive treatment, and excluding other possible causes. The clinical manifestations of PNF result from a lack of functional liver parenchyma necessary to sustain life and the development of necrotic tissue within the body. Despite the varying definition of PNF, the hallmark of this syndrome manifests as hyperbilirubinemia, elevated transaminases, metabolic acidosis, severe coagulopathy, lactic acidosis, absence of bile production, a need for pulmonary and hemodynamic support, hypoglycemia, acute renal failure, encephalopathy, and the absence of an identifiable surgical complication in the immediate period following reperfusion of the transplanted liver [37]. As PNF resides on a spectrum of graft dysfunction, distinguishing PNF from EAD can be difficult. Nevertheless, like any critically ill patient in the hospital, comprehensive organ support is needed. Patients with liver disease generally exist in a hyperdynamic state, defined as an increased heart rate and a low systemic vascular resistance due to peripheral/splanchnic vasodilation [49]. This state will persist with a nonfunctioning graft and can be further exacerbated by intraoperative fluid losses during transplantation. Therefore, aggressive fluid resuscitation, vasopressor support, and close hemodynamic monitoring are crucial [50].

The liver is responsible for clearing almost 70% of lactate from circulation with the remaining 30% removed by the kidneys [51]. In the setting of severe metabolic acidosis secondary to hepatic allograft failure, initiating early veno-venous hemofiltration can ameliorate the detrimental effects and help manage electrolyte fluxes associated with metabolic dysfunction [52]. Hepatic allograft dysfunction also increases the susceptibility to sepsis, and sepsis increases the susceptibility to organ hypoperfusion [53]. Most transplant recipients will not have a known infection prior to undergoing a liver transplant. However, because the liver is a crucial piece of the immune system, patients with evolving allograft dysfunction are increasingly susceptible to infectious insults. Therefore, initiation of broad-spectrum antibacterial and anti-fungal agents are recommended in patients suspected of evolving graft dysfunction [54]. The liver also secretes essential coagulation factors for hemostasis that are not produced by the injured liver in graft dysfunction. During transplantation there is an increased release of tissue plasminogen activator (TPA) from the graft endothelium, as such, hyperfibrinolysis may occur posing a significant hemodynamic threat to the patient in the setting of fibrinolysis and inability of the new graft to secrete coagulation factors from primary failure [55]. Therefore, aggressive support with blood products and monitoring the response with thromboelastograph is a staple in the post-transplant management and critical to distinguishing EGD that will recover from PNF that may warrant re-listing.

Although donor and recipient risk factors play a primary role in the evolution of PNF, there is increasing awareness of an accumulated risk of transplantation and the variety of factors involved compound the risk and make distinguishing cause and effect difficult. The liver is a complex organ with many vital functions that act in concert with the cardiovascular, renal, gastrointestinal, and many other systems throughout the body. Thus, the concept of donor risk factors, allograft characteristics, recipient features, procurement technique, preservation method, and implantation procedure likely all play a role in the development of PNF and overall success of liver transplantation [54]. For example, a recipient with multiple comorbidities who is more unwell, nutritionally deficient, deconditioned, is likely to be at an increased risk of transplant related complications, including PNF. Particularly when a suboptimal allograft is utilized.

Despite advances in transplantation operative techniques, post-surgical care, and immunosuppression, the presence of PNF remains an emergency with a high mortality rate without re-transplantation. In the United States, the Organ Procurement and Transplantation Network (OPTN) defines PNF based on the presence of specific laboratory derangement within 7 days of transplantation [56]. Although the definition of PNF varies in the literature and must continually be evaluated for improvements, this specific definition by OPTN is the most crucial as it allows for patient re-listing. Patients who are diagnosed with PNF are re-listed for re-transplantation with the highest priority (status 1A). To assign a candidate adult status 1A, the candidate's transplant hospital must submit a Liver Status 1A Justification Form to the OPTN Contractor. The transplant hospital must submit laboratory results for all required tests from the same blood draw taken 24 hours to 7 days after the transplant.

The achilles heel of transplantation is the organ shortage and our ability to effectively predict allograft recovery and function following donation and implantation. One strategy aimed at improving liver transplant outcomes is machine perfusion. In a meta-analysis by Zhang et al. [57] comparing hypothermic oxygenated perfusion (HOPE) technique with classic cold storage found a lower incidence of graft dysfunction in the perfusion group. Additionally, a randomized prospective trial from Nasralla et al. [58] compared normothermic machine perfusion (NMP) with classic static cold storage and found graft dysfunction was significantly decreased (10.1% to 29.9%) in the perfusion group. Although these studies evaluated outcomes of graft dysfunction and not specifically PNF, the results are promising and a component of optimizing the transplant process. With the growing demand for organs, non-heart-beating donors also known as donors after cardiac death (DCD) are being utilized with greater frequency. Once thought to be unsuitable for transplantation due to the nature of inadequate perfusion of organs after cardiac death, their use is becoming more common. Still, large multicenter studies show worse outcomes with the use of organs from DCD donors [59]. However, literature on rates of PNF in DCD recipients is mixed with some showing a higher incidence of primary nonfunction from DCD grafts [59], and other studies not showing any increase in PNF [60, 61]. With literature still pointing to worse outcomes in DCD recipients, having similar rates of PNF does not provide enthusiasm for regular use of DCD livers and is an area of continued research. That said, technological advances utilizing warm perfusion and normothermic regional organ recovery may increase opportunities to utilize DCD livers to bridge the growing disparity between organ supply and demand.

There are many factors at play during a transplant procedure and assessing each individual part is necessary to discover liver protective strategies and improve outcomes. A study from Korea compared the use of alprostadil after intravenous administration versus portal vein administration speculating an anti-inflammatory benefit for patients undergoing liver transplant and found lower aminotransferase levels on post-op day 1 in the portal vein injection group. Unfortunately, this study did not directly assess graft dysfunction or PNF rates [62]. The potential benefit of improved allograft perfusion of alprostadil to mitigate dysfunction has also not been born out. Another study using N-acetylcysteine during liver transplantation, a well-known compound used for liver toxicity found a significantly better profile of anti-inflammatory cytokines post-operatively [63]. However, another study by Gómez-Gavara et al. [64] found no differences in the incidence of EAD between a group receiving N-acetylcysteine versus control. Intraoperative modulation of blood flow has also been studied for varying protective strategies. Ischemic preconditioning (IP) by inducing periods of controlled ischemia in the donor graft has shown benefit. Amador et al. [65] assessed this strategy using the Pringle maneuver and found PNF was less common in the treatment group, but the results were not statistically significant. In a systematic review and meta-analysis by Robertson Et al. [66] evaluating IP in liver transplant donors, they found a beneficial effect of IP intervention with lower aminotransferase activity postoperative, decreased postoperative mortality, lower risk of PNF, and reduced need for re-transplantation. Although again, these results did not reach statistical significance.

In the end, if a hepatic allograft experiences primary non-function without signs of clinical improvement, re-transplantation is the only solution for that failed graft. Outcomes for re-transplantation are still poor with recent data showing 30 day and 1 year survival rates of 54–73% and 51–66%, respectively [33, 67, 68]. Additionally, re-transplantation of another allograft in the setting of PNF has been shown as an independent risk factor for PNF in the new allograft [69]. Decisions to undergo re-transplantation are difficult and require experienced transplant teams to evaluate graft dysfunction with poor recovery and mortality without re-transplantation. This decision-making process is unlikely to become easier but the factors and protective strategies to optimize risk and management of primary nonfunction have significantly improved and need continued study **Tables 1** and **2**.

Donor Factor
Age > 40 years
Female
African American Race
Cause of Death
Trauma
Stroke
Anoxia
Partial/Split
Donation after Cardiac Death
HBcAb Positive
HCV Positive
Sodium >170 mEq/L
Donor Height > 170 cm

Table 1.
Descriptive donor risk index (DRI) parameters.

Candidates may be assigned status 1A if all the following conditions are met:

1. The candidate has a life expectancy without a liver transplant of less than 7 days.
2. Primary non-function of a transplanted whole liver within 7 days of transplant, with an aspartate aminotransferase (AST) greater than or equal to 3000 U/L and at least one of the following:
   a. International normalized ratio (INR) greater than or equal to 2.5
   b. Arterial pH less than or equal to 7.30
   c. Venous pH less than or equal to 7.25
   d. Lactate greater than or equal to 4 mmol/L
3. Primary non-function within 7-days of transplant of a transplanted liver segment from a deceased or living donor, evidenced by at least one of the following:
   a. INR greater than or equal to 2.5
   b. Arterial pH less than or equal to 7.30
   c. Venous pH less than or equal to 7.25
   d. Lactate greater than or equal to 4 mmol/L

Table 2.
Candidate definition for re-transplantation.

2. Hepatic artery thrombosis in emergencies after liver transplant

Graft function following orthotopic liver transplantation relies on arterial perfusion. Despite improvements in anastomotic techniques and surgical grafting, vascular complications following solid organ transplant are not uncommon. Serious vascular complications can occur in the hepatic artery, hepatic vein, portal vein, and inferior vena cava following a liver transplant. The most common and severe vascular complication is hepatic artery thrombosis (HAT), resulting in absent arterial blood flow that can lead to graft failure, and loss requiring re-transplantation [70–72]. Other less severe complications include hepatic artery stenosis, aneurysm, and steal syndromes [71, 73, 74]. Although any vascular complication represents a significant pathology that must be promptly assessed, evaluated, and treated, this review will focus on HAT as it represents a true surgical emergency following liver transplantation.

Following orthotopic liver transplantation, HAT can be divided into early and late forms, with early HAT (E-HAT) generally having a severe clinical course, whereas late HAT (L-HAT) can be asymptomatic and better tolerated [75]. The definition of E-HAT versus L-HAT remains unclear with a cut off in the literature ranging from two weeks to 100 days [76, 77]. However, most of the literature addressing HAT specifies E-HAT to be within 21 days to one month [78–80]. Due to the discrepancy in definition within the literature, establishing consistent incidence rates, risk factors, and treatment regimens is difficult. Overall, the incidence of HAT (both E-HAT and L-HAT) ranges from 2.9–9% in adult patients [70, 75, 81], and from 4 to 26% in pediatric patients [82, 83]. The difference in incidence rates among adults and children is partly due to the theorized pathophysiology of HAT, that is the smaller caliber of donor and/or recipient arteries in the pediatric population increases the likelihood of occlusive thrombus [83]. A study by Mourad et al. [78] of 1487 orthotopic liver transplants found the incidence of E-HAT to be 2% and L-HAT 4.8%, and a systematic review by Bekker et al. [75] of 21,822 liver transplantations described only E-HAT and found an incidence of 4.4%. It is difficult to interpret which etiology of HAT, early or late, occurs more frequently but overall, HAT is the most common arterial complication in liver transplantation, and although still rare in practice, this dreaded complication is associated with mortality rates of up to 55% and the need for re-transplantation approaches 83% [70].

The pathophysiology and underlying causes of HAT remain a matter of debate and is likely multifactorial. Whereas the native liver can withstand major obstruction to its arterial blood supply due to flow through collaterals arising from the intrahepatic left and right arteries, superior mesenteric artery, inferior phrenic artery, left gastric artery, and arteries of the omentum and duodenum, the transplanted liver relies on the main hepatic artery during the early post-transplant recovery [37, 78]. Some studies have described the anatomical and pathological findings in both E-HAT and L-HAT. E-HAT has been shown to cause massive ischemic injury to hepatocytes and bile duct epithelial cells, causing graft dysfunction, bile leaks, abscess formation, infection, sepsis, and death [79, 84]. Compared to L-HAT, which has been described as a more insidious process resulting in biliary tract complications that can also cause bile leaks and abscess formation when severe [70, 78]. Given this natural history of disease processes, E-HAT has been associated with a 33.3% higher mortality than L-HAT, likely due to widespread necrosis leading to sepsis in the immunocompromised host [75, 85].

Surgical technique, hemodynamic fluxes, immunologic factors, reperfusion injury, and hypercoagulability have all been implicated in the evolution of HAT [76, 86]. In the realm of vascular medicine, Virchow's triad of thromboembolic disease: hypercoagulable state, venous stasis, and blood vessel damage describe the underpinnings of clotting within the body [87]. In orthotopic liver transplantation, patients commonly experience all three of these pillars during the creation of the arterial anastomosis. Thus, surgical factors are critical to describing HAT [37, 88].

As surgeons, the technical handling during transplantation is one factor that can be directly assessed and constantly improved. Arterial torsion, anastomotic stenoses, and small caliber vessels can all impact anastomotic success. To decrease the rates of these complications, meticulous arterial reconstruction and the use of microsurgical techniques using microscopes or loupes has long been stressed for vascular anastomoses [89, 90]. A systematic review by Pinto et al. [80] showed liver transplants using continuous 7–0 or 8–0 polypropylene suture for arterial anastomosis presented a 6.5% prevelence of HAT whereas interrupted suture dropped the prevalence to 2.5%. Similarly, a study by Zhao et al. [91] showed microvascular surgical technique for arterial anastomosis in liver transplants using interrupted suture and 3.5x loupes obtained a HAT prevalence of 1.4%. Additionally, Bekker et al. [75] and Salvalaggio et al. [92] have described lower volume transplant centers have an increased risk of HAT. Suggesting that clinical experience and expertise play a major role in transplantation outcomes and proficiency in these techniques is critical to limiting transplant complications.

Some studies have associated the number and type of anastomoses as risks for HAT. Both Mourad et al. [78] and Piscaglia et al. [93] found increasing number of arterial anastomoses significantly increased the risk of E-HAT. This inherently makes sense within the construct of Virchow's Triad, as more manipulation of the vessel endothelium disrupts the usual activating and inhibiting factors of coagulation, platelet adhesion, thrombosis, and may lead to a greater propensity to clot. Furthermore, two multivariate analyses showed that the use of arterial conduits had an increased incidence of E-HAT (15%) compared to a group without arterial conduit use (2%) [86, 94]. Additionally, the type of anastomosis has been shown to impact rates of HAT. Bilik et al. reported HAT in up to 25% of transplants that used donor iliac artery interposition grafts to the aorta and 6.6% with native hepatic artery use [95]. In a study by Stange et al. [70] using the donor hepatic artery with an aortic patch or the donor celiac trunk for arterial anastomosis, HAT occurred in 1.7% and 5.2%, respectively. A similar result was obtained with the infrarenal interposition graft (5.6%) and anastomosis between donor aortic patch or celiac trunk and recipient splenic artery (0.8%). However, a significantly greater incidence of HAT (10.4%) was observed if a supraceliac graft interposition was performed. Reduced size liver grafts (non-whole) have shown to have a reduced incidence of HAT in pediatric populations, likely due to the preferential use of adult grafts with relatively larger vessel diameters [96–98]. However, in the adult population grafting based on size is a less likely option and due to anatomic variability, certain grafts will inevitably pose greater challenges. Current literature may serve as a basis for preferential anastomosis use, but clinical experience and expertise should continue to guide surgical technique for liver transplantation.

While surgical technique is commonly implicated in the evolution of HAT, many non-operative factors increase the risk of peri-transplant thrombosis. Studies have shown that having multiple transplants, a recipient/donor weight ratio > 1.25, biopsy-proven rejection within 1 week of transplant, arterial anastomosis to an old conduit, and Cytomegalovirus (CMV) seronegative patients receiving an allograft from CMV seropositive donors have all been found to be risk factors for developing E-HAT [86]. CMV status is a particular area of interest as it is estimated that the global seroprevalence of CMV is 83% [99], and multiple studies have confirmed this increase in risk of HAT with a CMV seropositive donor to a CMV seronegative recipient [75, 100, 101]. The theory behind CMV's role in HAT is through the viral ability to infect endothelial cells in the context of surgical manipulation of vessels and endothelial damage increasing the propensity for clotting once tissue factor is exposed producing a procoagulant response [100].

In Comparison, risk factors for L-HAT have been described less commonly in the literature. Likely due to the varying definitions and confounding variables at play with long term follow-up of these patients. However, L-HAT does have some specific risk factors within the literature, female donor to male recipient, Hepatitis-C seropositive, tobacco use, and re-transplant for E-HAT have all been implicated as risk factors [102, 103]. Additionally, Levy et al. described that ongoing smoking after a liver transplant was associated with HAT [104]. Donor age has also been described as a possible risk factor for developing HAT, however the literature is still discordant and in a time of increasing need for organs creates a difficult dilemma. Margarit et al. showed that donor age was a significant predisposing factor for the development of biliary complications secondary to L-HAT in adult liver transplant patients [105]. In the pediatric transplant population, Sieder et al. reported that a lower Donor/Recipient age ratio (D/R Ratio) was a risk factor for developing HAT [106], and while older donors are believed to be at increased risk for HAT in adult transplant recipients, Oh et al. [107] did not find that advanced donor age increased the risk of thrombosis.

The clinical presentation of HAT is variable and differs between E-HAT and L-HAT. Pinna et al. [108] postulated that one third of arterial thrombi are asymptomatic, one third lead to ischemic syndromes but are not life threatening, and one third cause parenchymal necrosis leading to rapid death if not rectified promptly, and this notion is generally well accepted in clinical outcomes. The bile ducts of the hepatobiliary system are solely dependent on blood supply from the hepatic artery, thus manifestations of HAT generally present with a biliary tract damage [75, 78]. In the early postoperative period, E-HAT usually presents with fevers, abdominal pain, elevated transaminases, and elevated bilirubin levels [37, 109]. Due to the early complete occlusion of the hepatic artery in E-HAT, ischemic changes in the liver and biliary system allow translocation of bacteria from the portal circulation leading to sepsis and septic shock [37, 109]. On the other hand, L-HAT, which is less well described in the literature, has tremendous variability in presentation. Multiple studies have described that L-HAT may be asymptomatic and only discovered incidentally on imaging [78, 102]. Improvements in vascular imaging has demonstrated the formation of collateral blood flow leading to improved outcomes in cases of L-HAT and, as a result, asymptomatic arterial thrombosis of the hepatic artery that is found incidentally [110, 111]. However, the timing for such angiogenesis is variable but estimated to start within two weeks to four months [111]. If not entirely asymptomatic, L-HAT can present with fevers, cholangitis, bacteremia as well as many non-specific symptoms like back pain, shoulder pain, and fatigue [102, 103].

In the early postoperative period, surveillance for HAT differs considerably based on institutional protocols. Outside of the postoperative period, the evaluation of HAT becomes more ambiguous due to variable follow up and routine versus symptom-based screening [75]. The mainstay of screening in the modern era is Doppler Ultrasonography (US), that is a proven noninvasive modality to investigate hepatic artery patency [112, 113]. Doppler US is cost-effective, noninvasive, and relatively fast but is operator dependent and may vary due to individual patient differences. Thus, catheter angiography remains the gold standard to diagnose HAT [114]. More recently, a multidetector CT angiography can also be used as a fast, noninvasive way to test arterial patency with good sensitivity and specificity and may be used as an alternative [114].

Prompt evaluation and imaging is necessary when HAT is suspected in the post-transplant patient. With advances in interventional radiology and minimally invasive techniques, the treatment of HAT has changed. Graft reconstruction, surgical thrombectomy, and radiology guided thrombolysis are all available techniques to resolve HAT. However, with diagnosed E-HAT (creating graft dysfunction and severe illness by definition), re-transplantation remains the gold standard for definitive treatment [78]. Multiple studies have reported that prompt revascularization (either surgical or radiological) decreases the need for re-transplantation in cases of E-HAT [108, 115, 116]. recent endovascular advancements, modalities such as intra-arterial thrombolysis, percutaneous transluminal angioplasty (PTA), and stent placement have been found to be effective and suitable for treatment of HAT [101, 117]. In 1989, Hidalgo et al. [118] reported the first successful cases of intra-arterial thrombolysis (IAT) for patients with L-HAT. These thrombolytic agents such as Tissue Plasminogen Activator (TPA) and Urokinase, convert plasminogen to plasmin that cleaves fibrin strands within a thrombus leading to its dissolution and their use is theorized to be better in fresh clots due to the high-water content and relatively poor fibrin matrix [74, 119]. However, unlike the well-established treatment algorithm for strokes, there is no consensus on the timing for use of these thrombolytic agents in HAT [117]. Dissolving a clot within the hepatic artery using a thrombolytic agent only temporizes the problem, as the underlying issue of clot formation has already occurred and must be addressed. In a study by Yang et al. [120] 62% of patients that underwent IAT for HAT subsequently had to undergo PTA with or without stenting to treat the pathology. For cases of E-HAT, revascularization attempts have a reported success rate of approximately 50%, with 30.3% of those then undergoing re-transplantation [75].

Traditionally, re-transplantation has been the primary treatment for HAT, with 53.1% of cases of E-HAT undergoing re-transplantation as the primary treatment in a systematic review [78]. In another study by Duffy et al. [88] 71% of E-HAT and 51% of L-HAT cases had to undergo re-transplantation. A retrospective analysis of 4000 consecutive transplants from the University of Pittsburgh showed that HAT was the indication for nearly one-third of the re-transplants performed at that institution [121]. The overall 1-year graft survival rate for re-transplantation after E-HAT is approximately 50%, while other vascular complications have graft survival rates up to 86% [122]. Re-transplantation is restricted by a limited donor pool and this disparity will likely continue to grow in the future. Urgent revascularization for HAT, offers the opportunity to prevent the need for re-transplantation but the success rate is still highly variable and likely only most beneficial in cases of early detection [75, 123]. Given the challenges we all face with organ allocation, we do recommend attempting early revascularization when arterial thrombosis is identified. Our preferred approach is creating an arterial conduit with donor iliac artery from an infra-renal location (**Figure 1a-c**). Other than insuring adequate iliac conduit is recovered during every liver recovery, maintaining appropriate orientation to prevent twisting and torsion during its creation and tunneling is critical to successful revascularization.

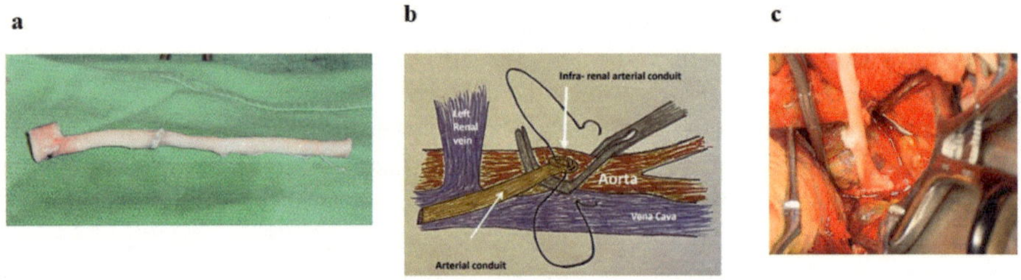

Figure 1.
a. Donor iliac artery. b. Infra-renal arterial conduit. c. Donor iliac artery arterial conduit.

Current recommendations rely on clinical experience and expertise with a great deal of institutional variability. It is recommended to integrate newer, minimally invasive modalities first when available, before proceeding to surgical thrombectomy, revascularization or re-transplantation due to the increased risks of reoperation in the early postoperative period and limited organ pool [70, 75, 116].

3. Portal vein thrombosis in emergencies after liver transplant

Portal Vein Thrombosis (PVT) is a well-known sequela of chronic liver disease, particularly in well-established cirrhosis [124]. With more than 60% of all liver transplants being performed for cirrhosis and cirrhosis being present in over 90% of cases of liver transplantation for hepatocellular carcinoma, PVT is a common finding during pre-transplant evaluation, intraoperative procedure, or as a complication following transplantation [124–126]. Once regarded as a contraindication to liver transplantation, PVT represents a common issue in cirrhotics and an increasingly common complication for transplant surgeons to manage [127]. PVT can be further classified based on anatomical or functional development, and multiple studies have described classification systems for the various etiologies of PVT [128–137].

PVT can be clinically insignificant and asymptomatic or become a true surgical emergency. Although it is not the most common vascular complication observed after orthotopic liver transplantation, it represents an important concern, especially given its context in the setting of the ever-increasing incidence of cirrhosis. It is important to note that much of the literature surrounding PVT is not in the context of transplant surgery, and clinicians will be presented with PVT primarily outside of the operating room. This review will discuss the prevalence, pathophysiology, risk factors, presentation and management of PVT when confronted during the perioperative period of an orthotopic liver transplant.

The prevalence of PVT varies throughout the literature, and incidence rates have been increasing in recent years due, in part, to improved diagnostic imaging [138]. Historically, the prevalence of PVT was 1–16% [124, 139–141], but with more screening and improved diagnostics, PVT may be diagnosed in up to 35% of cases in some series [138, 142]. It is important to note that the prevalence of PVT rises with the degree of liver damage, and with the development of hepatocellular carcinoma, incidence rates increase to 10% -40% [138, 143, 144]. Furthermore, studies have estimated that among all cases of PVT, cirrhosis is the underlying cause in 22% - 28% of cases PVT is often asymptomatic [126, 145]. As such, the frequency may still be underestimated in the current literature. PVT can be occlusive (or complete) or non-occlusive (or partial), and centers may differentiate their reporting to include both types or only to include occlusive thromboses as a case of PVT, further complicating the true prevalence [146]. Notably, the prevalence of newly discovered PVT after liver transplantation ranges from 1 to 5% and occurs more frequently in split grafts than in whole grafts [147].

The pathophysiology of PVT can be categorized into local and systemic factors. The portal venous system is a high flow, but low-pressure system that is prone to thrombus formation as a result of changes in the local environment from hepatobiliary factors such as the evolution of portal hypertension and inflammation from hepatocyte injury increasing the local resistance to flow. Various systemic factors also lead to PVT, such as inherited and acquired thrombophilic disorders, cancers, medications, and autoimmune disorders [128, 148]. Similar to the pathophysiology of HAT, the underlying causes of PVT can be contextualized within Virchow's Triad of thromboembolic disease (**Table 3**): hypercoagulable state, venous stasis, and blood vessel/endothelial cell damage that describe the underpinnings of clotting within the body [87]. Literature is consistent that at the origin of PVT, one or more factors of Virchow's Triad are usually present [149, 150].

First, the evolution of cirrhosis results in a stiff, fibrotic liver and these changes in the liver parenchyma increase the resistance to portal vein blood flow resulting in venous stasis, and increasing the propensity for the development of PVT [139, 145, 151]. A study by Zocco et al. [152] demonstrated that portal flow velocity is the most important predictive factor to the development of PVT and estimated that a flow of <15 cm/s on Doppler Ultrasound evaluation was associated with PVT. Additionally, splanchnic vasodilation from portal hypertension and "steal" effects from portosystemic shunting aid in developing venous stasis and reduced portal flow velocity [153, 154].

Second, the development of a hypercoagulable state known to be associated with underlying liver disease, and a variety of other prothrombotic states with the most obvious being malignancies like hepatocellular carcinoma, and common disorders such as Prothrombin gene G20210A mutations and Factor V Leiden are increasingly

Hypercoagulability:
• Factor V Leiden
• Prothrombin G20210A Gene mutation
• Protein C deficiency
• Protein S deficiency
• Antithrombin deficiency
• Malignancy/Neoplasm
• Hyperhomocysteinemia
• Non-alcoholic steatohepatitis (NASH), Non-alcoholic Fatty Liver Disease (NAFLD)
• Pregnancy
• Oral contraceptives
• Sepsis
Endothelial Cell Injury:
• Trauma
• Prior surgery
• Sclerotherapy
• Vascular manipulation, intravascular procedures
• Chemical irritation
• Radiation
• Infection
Venous Stasis:
• Cirrhosis
• Portal hypertension
• Beta Blockers

Table 3.
Virchow's triad of thromboembolic disease and factors relating to portal vein thrombosis.

associated with PVT in the literature [124, 155, 156]. In a study of patients with cirrhosis, a significant increase in factor VIII and D-dimer levels was observed in those with advanced cirrhosis, suggesting another intrinsic feature of the disease processes that increases the propensity to clot [157, 158]. Another study by Tripodi et al. [159] demonstrated that factor II, antithrombin, and protein C levels decrease progressively from Child-Turcotte-Pugh (CTP) class A to C. Furthermore, Non-alcoholic steatohepatitis (NASH) has been implicated as an independent risk factor for the development of PVT as it is associated with an increase in plasminogen activator inhibitor and reduced levels of protein C, further disrupting the clotting balance within the body [160, 161].

Finally, endothelial cell injury through trauma, surgical manipulation, radiation, chemical irritants, infection, and local inflammation round out common variables present in the patient with chronic liver disease presenting for primary transplantation that inherently drives clotting and the development of PVT [138, 162, 163]. Although Virchow's Triad establishes a reasonable basis for describing PVT, the underlying pathophysiology is likely multifactorial. Like prior topics in organ transplantation, multiple risk factors are crucial to the pathophysiology of any event.

Risk factors for the development of PVT are heterogeneous in the literature and most not validated, but many studies have attempted to describe various clinical parameters associated with PVT. Major risk factors for PVT are progressive liver disease severity, portal hypertension, obesity, metabolic syndrome, and NASH [146, 164]. More recently, a predictive model for PVT risk (**Table 4**) was developed with ten recipient characteristics identifying individuals at risk of developing PVT within 12 months of liver transplantation with good predictive value. These characteristics included African American ethnicity, age, diabetes, chronic hepatitis C, hepatocellular carcinoma, Hispanic ethnicity, MELD score, moderate/severe ascites, NASH, and TIPS procedure [165]. That same study found NASH to be a strong predictor of PVT risk in liver transplant candidates, which is significant given the epidemic of obesity and NASH that is now one of the leading indications for liver transplantation [166, 167]. Another study among 22,291 liver transplant recipients found that recipients with reported PVT were significantly older, more likely to be Caucasian, and had significantly higher MELD score at the time of transplant [146].

Occlusive PVT is known to complicate liver transplant procedures and is associated with a significant increase in mortality rates. Additionally, it is well established that PVT can lead to increased bleeding complications, hepato-hydrothorax, and other portal hypertensive-related complications. As such, patients with PVT awaiting liver transplantation may have a higher risk of significant morbidity and mortality [168, 169]. However, at this time, the presence of PVT is not incorporated into the major criterion for hepatic allograft allocation; therefore, the clinical expertise of the transplant team is heavily relied on when deciding to proceed with transplantation. Currently, screening for PVT is recommended during hepatocellular carcinoma screening for all potential transplant candidates [170].

Although the clinical presentation of PVT is variable and often asymptomatic in chronic cases, in the perioperative period for orthotopic liver transplantation, an acute PVT occlusion may develop with abdominal pain, ascites, splenomegaly, variceal

PVT RI = 0.335*NASH +0.095*MELD score + 0.126*Moderate/severe ascites +0.028*age (years) - 0.261*African American Race

Table 4.
Portal vein thrombosis risk index(RI) equation [165].

bleeding, and hepatic dysfunction [124, 128]. Patients with chronic PVT that develop symptoms often develop variceal bleeding due to worsening portal hypertension [124]. The diagnosis of PVT requires abdominal imaging to assess portal vein patency. The most common initial approach is doppler ultrasonography, with a reported overall sensitivity of 89–93% and specificity of 92–99% [171, 172]. Bubble contrast techniques can also improve ultrasound assessment [173]. If suggestive of PVT, abdominal computed tomography (CT) scans should be obtained where the classic features of acute PVT show hyperattenuating material in the portal vein and, with contrast injection, may show a lack of luminal enhancement during the arterial phase [174]. Comparatively, a chronic PVT is characterized by the presence of a portal cavernoma but may be more challenging to evaluate due to the evolution of collateral blood flow [175, 176]. Finally, improved magnetic resonance imaging (MRI) and CT angiography have 100% and 90% sensitivity and 98% and 99% specificity, respectively [172, 177], but transcatheter portal venography remains the gold standard diagnostic modality [37].

Adequate portal inflow is necessary for hepatic allograft survival. As such, PVT was long considered an absolute contraindication to liver transplantation [127]. The first successful liver transplantation in a patient with PVT was reported by Shaw et al. [178] in 1985. Since then, improvements in surgical technique and medical management have allowed liver transplantation to occur more often in the setting of PVT. That said, the presence of extensive thromboses remains a technical challenge during liver transplants [179]. A meta-analysis by Zanetto et al. [180] showed that 30-day mortality was higher in recipients with an existing complete PVT than a partial PVT. More recently, a classification system and treatment algorithm for portal inflow reconstruction during liver transplantation was established by Bhangui et al. [181] for patients undergoing liver transplantation with non-malignant PVT. This study classified reconstruction as physiologic when the splanchnic blood flow could be redirected to the liver and non-physiologic when the absence of a surgically created or spontaneous shunt did not relieve portal hypertension and found improved outcomes for this tailored surgical strategy based on PVT and inflow anatomy during transplantation. Although the study is based on pre-existing PVT during liver transplantation, it represents specified information that may help direct surgical strategies to prevent complications of PVT postoperatively.

The management of PVT relies on the severity of symptoms, size and location of the thrombus, existing shunts within the graft, type, timing of anticoagulation, and alternative interventional strategies available and again is reliant on the clinical expertise of the transplant team. Generally, anticoagulation is the primary management of surgical and non-surgical-related PVT [153]. Current data suggests that anticoagulation and recanalization of the portal vein is associated with improved survival and reduced portal hypertension-related complications in acute PVT [182]. However, data has shown that longstanding and extensive PVT in patients with cirrhosis decreases the likelihood of recanalization [179, 183]. Assessment of different anticoagulants has been well documented in the literature for PVT in the setting of cirrhosis, and both Low-Molecular-Weight Heparin (LMWH) and Warfarin have been shown to be effective in preventing the progression of PVT [184]. The use of Direct Oral Anticoagulants (DOACs) for treating PVT is emerging but still limited. A study by Hanafy et al. [185] on rivaroxaban versus warfarin for the management of acute PVT found that patients taking rivaroxaban achieved a higher rate of recanalization of the portal vein with improved survival rates than the patients receiving warfarin. Although the study represents a randomized controlled trial, further study and evaluation against LMWH must be done to establish the use of DOACs in acute PVT.

When anticoagulation is ineffective, the risk of clinical decompensation is high. In these cases, using thrombolysis, thrombectomy, percutaneous angioplasty with or without stenting, and Transjugular Intrahepatic Portosystemic Shunt (TIPS) creation have emerged as viable modalities to treat PVT. The initial escalation in treatment is generally thrombolysis with or without thrombectomy. In a meta-analysis of 71 patients with acute non-cirrhotic and non-malignant PVT, recanalization with thrombolysis and thrombectomy of the portal vein was complete in 40.8% and partial in 45.1% [186]. Percutaneous transhepatic balloon angioplasty is a minimally invasive technique considered safe and effective treatment of PVT but is not recommended if thrombolysis or thrombectomy can be performed or thromboses is extensive as there is a low likelihood of resolution [131, 187]. The use of TIPS procedure has shown a 67% - 100% recanalization success in patients with PVT [188, 189]. TIPS access allows for larger caliber access and avoids the risks of hemoperitoneum associated with transhepatic or transsplenic access [190].

One meta-analysis has demonstrated that pre-existing PVT is associated with a 50% increase in 1-year mortality following liver transplantation. However, with an end-to-end porto-portal anastomosis, the outcomes are similar to patients without pre-existing PVT with one and 5-year survival rates from 84–86%, and 65–80%, respectively [153]. Our experience corroborates these findings. As such, when confronted with portal vein thrombosis in the recipient, our technique has been to re-establish portal flow with a conduit from the infra-mesocolic or infra-pancreatic superior mesenteric vein (SMV) (**Figure 2a** and **b**) to the donor portal vein using donor iliac vein (**Figure 3a** and **b**). Isolating an infra-pancreatic segment of SMV can be a technical challenge. In those cases where it is a prohibitive challenge, it may be more straight forward to isolate a segment below the infra-mesocolon although this may require a midline extension of the chevron incision. In a similar manner, when recipients develop post-transplant PVT, our most common approach has involved surgical thrombectomy with revision of the anastomosis with an iliac vein conduit when the subjective flow post thrombectomy is not robust. Once a segment of superior mesenteric vein has been isolated, maintaining appropriate orientation to prevent twisting and torsion during its creation and tunneling is critical to successful revascularization. All repairs or revisions are subsequently treated with anticoagulation.

When the PVT does not improve with thrombectomy, surgical revision and medical treatment, it may propagate and reach the mesenteric venules causing

a b

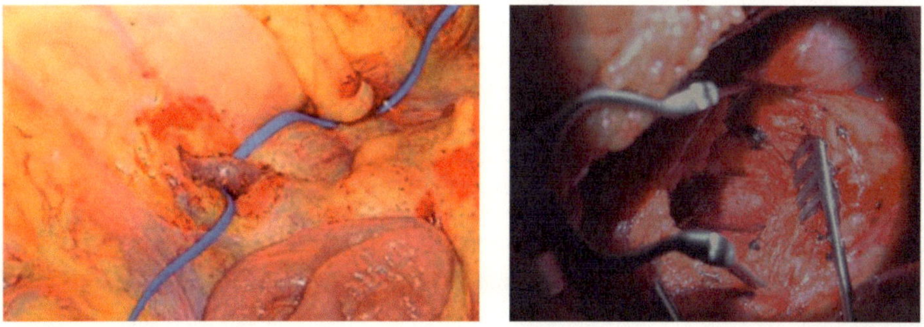

Figure 2.
a. Isolated superior mesenteric vein below the transverse mesocolon. b. Isolated superior mesenteric vein below the edge of the pancreas.

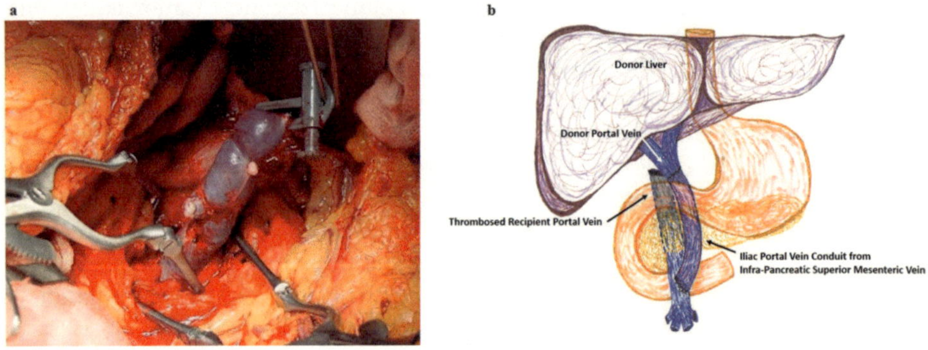

Figure 3.
a. Donor iliac vein conduit from the SMV. b. Donor iliac vein conduit from the SMV.

intestinal ischemia, placing the patient at an increased risk of peritonitis, sepsis, and death. However, the frequency of this is unclear in the current literature [191, 192]. Additionally, if acute PVT causes variceal bleeding, endoscopic sclerotherapy or banding may be required. It will sometimes suffice as a treatment regimen or must be combined with further definitive treatment modalities [116, 128]. With improved techniques, technology, and medical management for cases of acute PVT, re-transplantation following acute PVT is infrequently performed and not well described in the literature but remains an unfortunate alternative when acute PVT decompensates quickly leading to irreversible graft failure and thus must not be a forgotten alternative by the transplant clinician [193–195].

4. Outflow obstructions in emergencies after liver transplant

While there has been a great deal of evolution in many aspects of liver transplantation, the implantation of an orthotopic liver transplant has remined virtually unchanged since its inception with variations that have been introduced with live donor liver transplantation. Nevertheless, we are still forced to rely on native structures for allograft inflow and outflow. Variations and adaptations that are introduced by necessity during a transplant with nuances of each hepatectomy, size of an allograft, status of recipient vessels and implantation ultimately contribute to the complications that evolve following the procedure.

In the case of an orthotopic liver transplant, the diseased liver must be removed to allow implantation of a lifesaving organ. The hepatectomy can be performed expediently in some cases with cross clamping the supra-hepatic and infra-hepatic vena cava and excising the liver and retro-hepatic vena cava *en-bloc*. Alternatively, the liver may be, meticulously, dissected away from the vena cava and ultimately explanted at the level of the native hepatic veins leaving the recipient vena cava intact to preserve infra-diaphragmatic venous return. As such, the nature of the hepatectomy impacts how the allograft is implanted.

The hepatic allograft must, by necessity, drain through the recipient vena cava. This has classically been performed in one of three fashions. The first has utilized the standard implantation method which involves a bicaval anastomosis of the donor retro-hepatic vena-cava. This technique mandates temporary cessation of inferior vena-caval venous return while the donor supra-hepatic cava is sewn to the recipient supra-hepatic cava and the donor infra-hepatic cava is sewn to the recipient infra-hepatic cava. The second and possibly most common technique is referred to as the "piggyback" method. There are many variations on this theme. One variation during the "piggy-back" implantation involves creating a cloacae by dividing the common wall between the left and middle hepatic veins and the donor supra-hepatic vena cava is sewn to the cloacae in an end-to-side fashion [196]. Another commonly employed variation involves excising the middle and left hepatic veins at the junction with the vena cava and sewing the donor supra-hepatic vena cava in an end-to-side fashion to the caval orifice. The piggyback technique preserves the native cava but presents a technical challenge during the recipient hepatectomy. However, a significant hemodynamic benefit is realized with the preservation of preload from venous return and the avoidance of veno-venous bypass [197]. The third and least commonly employed technique involves a side-to-side cava-cavostomy. While the recipient vena cava is intact, it must be cross-clamped to perform the side-to-side cava-cavostomy. Therebye, losing the benefit of preload from subdiaphragmatic venous return. The benefit of this technique is that one creates a large outflow tract. As such, it should be clear that the transplant technique and manner in which the outflow tract was created is critical in any discussion of complications following liver transplantation involving venous outflow obstruction [198].

Venous outflow tract complications (VOC) involve the transplant hepatic veins or the inferior vena cava (IVC) and are relatively uncommon complications in clinical practice although the incidence rates vary throughout the literature. While infrequent, venous outflow obstruction can present serious complications including graft loss and death in the post-transplant period and thus is a crucial etiology to understand, prevent, and manage [199]. Outflow obstructions in the IVC following liver transplantation are uncommon and have been reported in 1.1% - 3.5% of cases [200–202]. Comparatively, hepatic vein outflow complication rates vary from 0.8% - 16.6% in the current literature with the higher end generally seen in partial split grafts compared to whole grafts, where split grafts show an increased frequency of venous outflow obstructions [203–211]. This discrepancy is likely due to the small caliber hepatic venous anastomosis to the IVC in split grafts and anastomotic distortion with buckling and twisting that can occur secondary to allograft growth after reperfusion [212–214]. Similarly, VOC is noted more frequently in pediatric liver transplants likely as a result of smaller diameter vessels and size mismatches from larger donor vessels to smaller recipient vessels increasing the reported incidence [209, 215–217].

The difference between conventional and piggyback technique regarding VOC varies in the literature. Traditionally, piggyback technique has shown a greater incidence of VOC with one study reporting VOC in 3% - 4% in adults and 5% - 15% in pediatrics compared to the conventional method where rates were < 2% [199, 218]. However, other studies have found no difference in VOC outcomes or reported improvements with the piggyback technique compared to the conventional [219, 220]. Interestingly, duplex ultrasonography post-transplant has not shown differences in hepatic venous flow between the two types of transplantation [220]. Furthermore, studies have attempted to evaluate the specific anastomotic landscape in relation to VOC and reports indicate end-to-side anastomosis of the graft to the mid and left hepatic veins leads to increased rates of VOC and that a side-to-side cavocavostomy improved this outcome [213]. Overall, the piggyback technique has shown validated improvements in surgical procedure and outcomes and remains the preferred method by many transplant programs. Regardless of procedure type, meticulous technique and microsurgical expertise are imperative to the success of outflow in the transplanted graft and transplant teams should continue the use of gold standard surgical techniques to avoid VOC regardless of transplant type.

Venous outflow tract complications (VOC) can be described as early or late, with the literature drawing the line at four weeks post-operatively [221, 222]. Early VOC are often viewed as a mechanical or technical complication of the transplant procedure, including rotation of the graft, twisting, kinking, tight sutures, compression, donor-recipient size mismatch, low recipient-to-donor body mass index ratio, or thrombosis [202, 221, 223–225]. Late VOC, occurring after four weeks post-transplant is generally thought to occur because of intimal hyperplasia or perivascular fibrosis and stenosis. Additionally, changes in the allograft size secondary to edema, fatty changes and inflammation can cause late changes in the anastomoses affecting the outflow tract [211, 221, 226–228]. Late VOC can be a recurrent process and is seen more frequently in patients with hypercoagulability and autoimmunity and are conditions that are exacerbated by endothelial cell damage during surgical anastomoses [229].

Patients with VOC present with manifestations of portal hypertension including refractory ascites, anasarca, renal dysfunction, and allograft dysfunction. The most commonly reported symptom of VOC after liver transplantation is refractory ascites [226, 230, 231]. When patients are transplanted with hypercoagulable conditions, recurrent Budd-Chiari syndrome should be suspected. If the patient presents with refractory ascites, anasarca and lower extremity edema, one should suspect involvement of IVC with stenosis and potentially thrombosis. Early signs of an outflow tract problem may be manifested biochemically with transaminitis, progressive cholestasis, and renal dysfunction [201, 202, 221, 222, 228, 232–234].

Patients suspected of having VOC after liver transplantation are generally evaluated with Doppler Ultrasonography (DUS) first, which may show a dampened, monophasic, or reversed waveform with elevated velocity across the stenosis in positive cases [201, 202, 235]. VOC is unlikely with the presence of a biphasic or triphasic waveform [236]. Additionally, finding reduced pulsatility is associated with hepatic vein stenosis [237]. The venous pulsatility index (PVI) was described in two studies and has shown a specificity of 95.7% for PVI < 0.45, which can be used to improve the specificity of DUS for VOC [238, 239]. Additionally, CT and MR angiography are appropriate diagnostic tools for VOC. CT imaging may reveal similar findings or contrast defects in the hepatic venous outflow tracts, and CT has demonstrated a better sensitivity and specificity for VOC when compared to DUS (97% vs. 87% and 86% vs. 68% respectively) [240]. Although invasive, the gold standard diagnostic technique is venography with manometry across the anastomosis. There is no accepted threshold of gradient flow to define VOC, but studies generally suggest 3–20 mmHg is clinically significant and deserves further investigation or intervention [201, 202, 235].

Given the underlying causes of early and late VOC are related to vessel caliber and flow dynamics, anticoagulation does not play a role in the treatment of this type of vascular obstruction. Evaluation and treatment of VOC is first approached with venography and manometry across the anastomosis with the benefit of simultaneous intervention. Vascular access through the right internal jugular vein (IJ) is preferred as the vein has a straight course and a clinically proven safety profile [241]. Alternatively, the left IJ and femoral vein can be used for access and, rarely, a transhepatic option allows access to the anastomotic dilemma [242, 243].

Since the advent of diverse and precise endovascular interventions, the primary treatment for VOC transitioned to endovascular approaches as opposed to surgical revisions. However, in the immediate perioperative period, surgical revision of venous anastomoses is preferred for definitive treatment [244]. Initial treatment of

VOC is venoplasty with balloons ranging from 8 to 14 mm in the hepatic veins and 12–18 mm in the IVC with the balloon size slightly oversized by 1–2 mm with respect to the diameter of the vein and inflation not exceeding 1–2 minutes [214, 222]. After sequential venoplasty, venography with manometry should be repeated to assess flow changes with one study suggesting a pressure gradient <3 mmHg achieving technical success [228]. Hepatic venoplasty has a complication rate < 1% and although there is a theoretical risk of vein rupture, no reported cases have been reported in the literature to date [228, 230, 245]. Technical success of improving flow across a venous anastomosis is high, but recurrence is common and occurs in approximately 55% of cases within 5 years necessitating repeated venoplasty and further intervention [214].

Vascular stenting in addition to angioplasty has shown a high degree of technical and clinical success in recent years. Retrospective data has shown 5-year patency rates of 72–94% and 10-year rates of 70–88% with even better short-term outcomes reaching 99–100% in multiple studies at 1 year [209, 246, 247]. Furthermore, clinical success rates with venous stenting have reached 83.3% at 5-years in pediatric VOC cases following liver transplantation [205]. Additionally, although the cases are small in number, some studies have shown high rates of stent patency up to 13.5 and 17 years [205, 248].

Stent selection in terms of stent type and size is critical and generally relies on clinical experience and expertise. The difference between balloon-expandable and self-expandable stents in the treatment of VOC is a matter of debate. A balloon-expandable stent has greater radial force compared to a self-expanding stent, but a self-expanding stent can elastically recover following compression and is thought to be more amenable to intravascular anatomy [249]. However, both types of stents have been used and described with successful long term patency rates. As such, this deliberation requires further investigation to establish a definitive approach [209, 228, 246]. Overall, stenting appears to be a superior intervention for long term patency in the management of VOC following liver transplantation compared to venoplasty alone. However, many still favor venoplasty prior to primary stent placement due to possible stent associated complications. Moreover, there are known risks associated with venoplasty and stenting a new anastomosis and stent placement is critical. Minimizing stent extension into the IVC helps decrease the risk of caval stenosis and facilitates re-intervention or future re-transplantation [227].

Stent occlusion is a feared risk with any form of intravascular stenting and the use of drug-eluting stents has been well defined for the treatment of coronary artery disease but has not been explored for VOC [250]. Stent migration is another severe complication of stent placement and can occur secondary to cardiac or repsiratory motion or occur spontaneously due to the dynamic anatomy of blood vessels. In three retrospective studies totaling 63 cases of stent placement following VOC after liver transplant, there were only two recorded cases of stent migration, and only one of those cases required surgical intervention [204, 205, 245]. Although rare in the current literature, stent related complications can occur. As such, appropriate selection and technical aptitude must be implored when deciding to stent in VOC.

Stenosis or occlusion of the vena cava or hepatic veins used to be associated with high rates of re-transplantation after failed surgical or radiologic interventions to relief VOC [231, 251]. However, given the advances in endovascular treatments and medical management, re-transplantation for VOC has become rare in the modern era with improvements in surgical thrombectomy, venoplasty, and stenting. And although VOC remains a relatively rare complications following orthotopic liver transplantation, it carries a significant risk of morbidity and mortality if not diagnosed and appropriately treated.

Liver transplantation has progressed since its inception. Medical management of patients with end stage liver diseases has improved allowing more patients to survive to a point where a liver transplant has become the next expected treatment. As such, more patients are waiting on the wait list for a liver transplant motivating transplant teams to push the boundaries and utilize what were once marginal organs for transplantation. In parallel, anesthetic management, surgical techniques, immunosuppression and postoperative care have improved considerably resulting in unbelievable success and outcomes we never thought would be achieved. These successes are often borne from tragedy that is a consequence of trial and error. New fields have emerged and are contributing significantly to our shared success in transplantation such as the evolution of Interventional Radiology and Transplant Oncology. As we push the envelope in our quest to save more lives, we will invariably encounter new and old complications, but our new multidisciplinary approach provides the advantage of better decision-making with higher quality, less morbid outcomes. Central to achieving the best possible outcomes is a collaborative participation of the multidisciplinary team members in an open discussion of all relevant medical, anatomical and surgical factors yielding optimal approaches to resolving each challenge.

Author details

Brian L. Shaw[1], Bill S. Majdalany[2] and Carlos E. Marroquin[3*]

1 Larner College of Medicine at The University of Vermont, USA

2 Larner College of Medicine and University of Vermont Medical Center, USA

3 East Carolina University Health, Greenville, North Carolina, USA

*Address all correspondence to: carlos.marroquin@ECUHealth.org

References

[1] Masior Ł, Grąt M. Primary nonfunction and early allograft dysfunction after liver transplantation. Digestive Diseases. 2022;**40**(6):766-776. DOI: 10.1159/000522052

[2] Ploeg RJ, D'Alessandro AM, Knechtle SJ, et al. Risk factors for primary dysfunction after liver transplantation—A multivariate analysis. Transplantation. 1993;**55**(4):807-813. DOI: 10.1097/00007890-199304000-00024

[3] Alonso IJ, Nutu A, García-Conde M, et al. Incidence and risk factors of primary non-function after liver transplantation using grafts from uncontrolled donors after circulatory death. Clinical Transplantation. 2020;**35**(1):e14134. DOI: 10.1111/ctr.14134

[4] Johnson SR, Alexopoulos SP, Curry MP, Hanto DW. Primary nonfunction (PNF) in the MELD era: An SRTR database analysis. American Journal of Transplantation. 2007;**7**(4):1003-1009. DOI: 10.1111/j.1600-6143.2006.01702.x

[5] Taner CB, Bathala V, Nguyen JH. Primary nonfunction in liver transplantation: A single-Center experience. Transplantation Proceedings. 2008;**40**(10):3566-3568. DOI: 10.1016/j.transproceed.2008.07.137

[6] Kemmer N, Secic M, Zacharias V, Kaiser TE, Neff G. Long-term analysis of primary nonfunction in liver transplant recipients. Transplantation Proceedings. 2007;**39**(5):1477-1480. DOI: 10.1016/j.transproceed.2006.11.012

[7] Al-Freah M, McPhail M, Dionigi E, et al. Improving the diagnostic criteria for primary liver graft nonfunction in adults utilizing standard and transportable laboratory parameters: An outcome-based analysis. American Journal of Transplantation. 2017;**17**(5):1255-1266. DOI: 10.1111/ajt.14230

[8] Mazariegos G, Molmenti EP, Kramer DJ. Early complications after ORTHOTOPIC liver transplantation. Surgical Clinics of North America. 1999;**79**(1):109-129. DOI: 10.1016/s0039-6109(05)70009-8

[9] Colina F, Lopez-Carreira M, Moreno E, et al. A clinopathologic review of 8 liver graft primary nonfunctions. PubMed. 1995;**42**(3):212-221. Available from: https://pubmed.ncbi.nlm.nih.gov/7590568

[10] Massip-Salcedo M, Roselló-Catafau J, Prieto J, Avíla MA, Peralta C. The response of the hepatocyte to ischemia. Liver International. Feb 2007;**27**(1):6-16. DOI: 10.1111/j.1478-3231.2006

[11] Peralta C, Jiménez-Castro MB, Gracia-Sancho J. Hepatic ischemia and reperfusion injury: Effects on the liver sinusoidal milieu. Journal of Hepatology. 2013;**59**(5):1094-1106. DOI: 10.1016/j.jhep.2013.06.017

[12] Ali JM, Davies S, Brais R, et al. Analysis of ischemia/reperfusion injury in time-zero biopsies predicts liver allograft outcomes. Liver Transplantation. 2015;**21**(4):487-499. DOI: 10.1002/lt.24072

[13] Itô T, Naini BV, Markovic D, et al. Ischemia-reperfusion injury and its relationship with early allograft dysfunction in liver transplant patients. American Journal of Transplantation. 2021;**21**(2):614-625. DOI: 10.1111/ajt.16219

[14] Feng S, Goodrich NP, Bragg-Gresham JL, et al. Characteristics associated with liver graft failure: The concept of a donor risk index. American Journal of Transplantation. 2006;**6**(4):783-790. DOI: 10.1111/j.1600-6143.2006.01242.x

[15] Merion RM, Goodrich NP, Feng S. How can we define expanded criteria for liver donors? Journal of Hepatology. 2006;**45**(4):484-488. DOI: 10.1016/j.jhep.2006.07.016

[16] Dutkowski P, Schlegel A, Slankamenac K, et al. The use of fatty liver grafts in modern allocation systems. Annals of Surgery. 2012;**256**(5):861-869. DOI: 10.1097/sla.0b013e318272dea2

[17] Bastos-Neves D, Salvalaggio PR, De Almeida MD. Risk factors, surgical complications and graft survival in liver transplant recipients with early allograft dysfunction. Hepatobiliary & Pancreatic Diseases International. 2019;**18**(5):423-429. DOI: 10.1016/j.hbpd.2019.02.005

[18] Sirivatanauksorn Y, Taweerutchana V, Limsrichamrern S, et al. Analysis of donor risk factors associated with graft outcomes in orthotopic liver transplantation. Transplantation Proceedings. 2012;**44**(2):320-323. DOI: 10.1016/j.transproceed.2011.12.031

[19] Kalisvaart M, Schlegel A, Umbro I, et al. The impact of combined warm ischemia time on development of acute kidney injury in donation after circulatory death liver transplantation. Transplantation. 2018;**102**(5):783-793. DOI: 10.1097/tp.0000000000002085

[20] Brokelman WJA, Stel A, Ploeg RJ. Risk factors for primary dysfunction after liver transplantation in the University of Wisconsin solution era. Transplantation Proceedings. 1999;**31**(5):2087-2090. DOI: 10.1016/s0041-1345(99)00270-5

[21] Monbaliu D, Pirenne J, Talbot D. Liver transplantation using donation after cardiac death donors. Journal of Hepatology. 2012;**56**(2):474-485. DOI: 10.1016/j.jhep.2011.07.004

[22] Houben P, Döhler B, Weiss KH, Mieth M, Mehrabi A, Süsal C. Differential influence of donor age depending on the indication for liver transplantation—A collaborative transplant study report. Transplantation. 2020;**104**(4):779-787. DOI: 10.1097/tp.0000000000002970

[23] De Boer J, Blok JJ, Putter H, et al. Optimizing the use of geriatric livers for transplantation in the Eurotransplant region. Liver Transplantation. 2019;**25**(2):260-274. DOI: 10.1002/lt.25353

[24] Lake JR, Shorr J, Steffen BJ, Chu A, Gordon RD, Wiesner RH. Differential effects of donor age in liver transplant recipients infected with hepatitis B, hepatitis C and without viral hepatitis. American Journal of Transplantation. 2005;**5**(3):549-557. DOI: 10.1111/j.1600-6143.2005.00741.x

[25] Cuende N, Grande L, Sanjuán FO, Cuervas-Mons V. Liver transplant with organs from elderly donors: Spanish experience with more than 300 liver donors over 70 years of age. Transplantation. 2002;**73**(8):1360. DOI: 10.1097/00007890-200204270-00033

[26] Houben P, Bormann E, Kneifel F, et al. How old is old? An age-stratified analysis of Elderly liver donors above 65. Journal of Clinical Medicine. 2022;**11**(13):3899. DOI: 10.3390/jcm11133899

[27] Busquets J, Xiol X, Figueras J, et al. The impact of donor age on liver

transplantation: Influence of donor age on early liver function and on subsequent patient and graft survival. Transplantation. 2001;**71**(12):1765-1771. DOI: 10.1097/00007890-200106270-00011

[28] Grande L, Matus D, Rimola A, Manyalic M, Cabrer C, García-Valdecasas JC, et al. Expanded liver donor age over 60 years for hepatic transplantation. Clinical Transplantation. 1998:297-301. PMID: 10503107

[29] Washburn WK, Johnson LB, Lewis WD, Jenkins RL. Graft function and outcome of older (???60 years) donor livers. Transplantation. 1996;**61**(7):1062-1066. DOI: 10.1097/00007890-199604150-00013

[30] Chavin KD, Yang S, Lin HK, et al. Obesity induces expression of uncoupling protein-2 in hepatocytes and promotes liver ATP depletion. Journal of Biological Chemistry. 1999;**274**(9):5692-5700. DOI: 10.1074/jbc.274.9.5692

[31] Adam R, Reynès M, Johann M, et al. The outcome of steatotic grafts in liver transplantation. PubMed. 1991;**23**(1 Pt 2):1538-1540. Available from: https://pubmed.ncbi.nlm.nih.gov/1989281

[32] Chu MJJ, Dare AJ, Phillips ARJ, Bartlett A. Donor hepatic steatosis and outcome after liver transplantation: A systematic review. Journal of Gastrointestinal Surgery. 2015;**19**(9):1713-1724. DOI: 10.1007/s11605-015-2832-1

[33] Kulik U, Lehner F, Klempnauer J, Borlak J. Primary non-function is frequently associated with fatty liver allografts and high mortality after re-transplantation. Liver International. 2017;**37**(8):1219-1228. DOI: 10.1111/liv.13404

[34] Cieślak B, Lewandowski Z, Urban M, Ziarkiewicz-Wróblewska B, Krawczyk M. Microvesicular liver graft steatosis as a risk factor of initial poor function in relation to suboptimal donor parameters. Transplantation Proceedings. 2009;**41**(8):2985-2988. DOI: 10.1016/j.transproceed.2009.08.019

[35] Westerkamp AC, De Boer MT, Van Den Berg AP, Gouw ASH, Porte RJ. Similar outcome after transplantation of moderate macrovesicular steatotic and nonsteatotic livers when the cold ischemia time is kept very short. Transplant International. 2014;**28**(3):319-329. DOI: 10.1111/tri.12504

[36] McCormack L, Petrowsky H, Jochum W, Müllhaupt B, Weber M, Clavien P. Use of severely steatotic grafts in liver transplantation. Annals of Surgery. 2007;**246**(6):940-948. DOI: 10.1097/sla.0b013e31815c2a3f

[37] Marroquin CE, Tuttle-Newhall JE, Collins BH, Kuo PC, Schroeder RA. Emergencies after liver transplantation. Seminars in Gastrointestinal Disease. 2003;**14**(2):101-110

[38] Totsuka E, Dodson F, Urakami A, et al. Influence of high donor serum sodium levels on early postoperative graft function in human liver transplantation: Effect of correction of donor hypernatremia. Liver Transplantation and Surgery. 1999;**5**(5):421-428. DOI: 10.1002/lt.500050510

[39] Olthoff KM, Kulik L, Samstein B, et al. Validation of a current definition of early allograft dysfunction in liver transplant recipients and analysis of risk factors. Liver Transplantation. 2010;**16**(8):943-949. DOI: 10.1002/lt.22091

[40] Markmann JF, Markmann JW, Markmann DA, et al. Preoperative

factors associated with outcome and their impact on resource use IN 1148 consecutive primary liver transplants. Transplantation. 2001;**72**(6):1113-1122. DOI: 10.1097/00007890-200109270-00023

[41] Farmer DG, Anselmo DM, Ghobrial RM, et al. Liver transplantation for fulminant hepatic failure. Annals of Surgery. 2003;**237**(5):666-676. DOI: 10.1097/01.sla.0000064365.54197.9e

[42] Weimann A, Braga M, Harsányi L, et al. ESPEN guidelines on enteral nutrition: Surgery including organ transplantation. Clinical Nutrition. 2006;**25**(2):224-244. DOI: 10.1016/j.clnu.2006.01.015

[43] Hine C, Harputlugil E, Zhang Y, et al. Endogenous hydrogen sulfide production is essential for dietary restriction benefits. Cell. 2015;**160**(1-2):132-144. DOI: 10.1016/j.cell.2014.11.048

[44] Pruim J, Van Woerden WF, Knol EF, et al. Donor data in liver grafts with primary non-function--a preliminary analysis by the European liver registry. PubMed. 1989;**21**(1 Pt 2):2383-2384. Available from: https://pubmed.ncbi.nlm.nih.gov/2652776

[45] Miyauchi T, Uchida Y, Kadono K, et al. Preventive effect of antioxidative nutrient-rich enteral diet against liver ischemia and reperfusion injury. Journal of Parenteral and Enteral Nutrition. 2018;**43**(1):133-144. DOI: 10.1002/jpen.1308

[46] Mitchell JR, Verweij M, Brand K, et al. Short-term dietary restriction and fasting precondition against ischemia reperfusion injury in mice. Aging Cell. 2010;**9**(1):40-53. DOI: 10.1111/j.1474-9726.2009

[47] Wang W, Xu S, Ren Z, Jiang J, Zheng S. Gut microbiota and allogeneic transplantation. Journal of Translational Medicine. 2015;**13**(1):40-53. DOI: 10.1186/s12967-015-0640-8

[48] Jacob M, Copley LP, Lewsey J, Gimson A, Rela M, Van Der Meulen J. Functional status of patients before liver transplantation As a predictor of Posttransplant mortality. Transplantation. 2005;**80**(1):52-57. DOI: 10.1097/01.tp.0000163292.03640.5c

[49] Møller S, Bendtsen F. The pathophysiology of arterial vasodilatation and hyperdynamic circulation in cirrhosis. Liver International. 2018;**38**(4):570-580. DOI: 10.1111/liv.13589

[50] Keegan MT, Kramer DJ. Perioperative care of the liver transplant patient. Critical Care Clinics. 2016;**32**(3):453-473. DOI: 10.1016/j.ccc.2016.02.005

[51] Vitin AA, Azamfirei L, Tomescu D, Lang JD. Perioperative Management of Lactic Acidosis in end-stage liver disease patient. Journal of Critical Care Medicine (Targu Mures). 2017;**3**(2):55-62. Published 2017 May 11. DOI: 10.1515/jccm-2017-0014

[52] Matuszkiewicz-Rowińska J, Wieliczko M, Małyszko J. Renal replacement therapy before, during, and after orthotopic liver transplantation. Annals of Transplantation. 2013;**18**:248-255. DOI: 10.12659/aot.883929

[53] Strnad P, Tacke F, Koch A, Trautwein C. Liver — Guardian, modifier and target of sepsis. Nature Reviews Gastroenterology & Hepatology. 2016;**14**(1):55-66. DOI: 10.1038/nrgastro.2016.168

[54] Hartog H, Hann A, Perera MTPR. Primary nonfunction of the liver allograft. Transplantation. 2021;**106**(1):117-128. DOI: 10.1097/tp.0000000000003682

[55] Hartmann M, Szalai C, Saner FH. Hemostasis in liver transplantation: Pathophysiology, monitoring, and treatment. World Journal of Gastroenterology. 2016;**22**(4):1541-1550. DOI: 10.3748/wjg.v22.i4.1541

[56] Organ Procurement & Transplantation Network. Available from: https://optn.transplant.hrsa.gov/ [Accessed: July 16, 2023]

[57] Zhang Y, Zhang Y, Zhang M, Ma Z, Wu S. Hypothermic machine perfusion reduces the incidences of early allograft dysfunction and biliary complications and improves 1-year graft survival after human liver transplantation. Medicine. 2019;**98**(23):e16033. DOI: 10.1097/md.0000000000016033

[58] Nasralla D, Coussios CC, Mergental H, et al. A randomized trial of normothermic preservation in liver transplantation. Nature. 2018;**557**(7703):50-56. DOI: 10.1038/s41586-018-0047-9

[59] Taylor R, Allen E, Richards J, et al. Survival advantage for patients accepting the offer of a circulatory death liver transplant. Journal of Hepatology. 2019;**70**(5):855-865. DOI: 10.1016/j.jhep.2018.12.033

[60] Martínez MP, Pérez BS, Díaz F, et al. Donation after cardiac death in liver transplantation: An additional source of organs with similar results to donation after brain death. Transplantation Proceedings. 2019;**51**(1):4-8. DOI: 10.1016/j.transproceed.2018.02.208

[61] Bohórquez H, Seal J, Cohen AJ, et al. Safety and outcomes in 100 consecutive donation after circulatory death liver transplants using a protocol that includes thrombolytic therapy. American Journal of Transplantation. 2017;**17**(8):2155-2164. DOI: 10.1111/ajt.14261

[62] Shin MJ, Song SH, Kim JM, et al. Effectiveness of intraportal prostaglandin E1 administration after liver transplantation. Transplantation Proceedings. 2012;**44**(2):500-504. DOI: 10.1016/j.transproceed.2012.01.070

[63] Santiago F, Bueno P, Olmedo C, et al. Effect of N-Acetylcysteine administration on intraoperative plasma levels of interleukin-4 and interleukin-10 in liver transplant recipients. Transplantation Proceedings. 2008;**40**(9):2978-2980. DOI: 10.1016/j.transproceed.2008.08.103

[64] Gómez-Gavara C, Moya-Herráiz Á, Hervás D, Pérez-Rojas J, Lahoz A, López-Andújar R. The potential role of efficacy and safety evaluation of N-Acetylcysteine administration during liver procurement. The NAC-400 single Center randomized controlled trial. Transplantation. 2021;**105**(10):2245-2254. DOI: 10.1097/tp.0000000000003487

[65] Amador A, Grande L, Marti J, et al. Ischemic pre-conditioning in deceased donor liver transplantation: A prospective randomized clinical trial. American Journal of Transplantation. 2007;**7**(9):2180-2189. DOI: 10.1111/j.1600-6143.2007.01914.x

[66] Robertson FP, Magill L, Wright GP, Fuller B, Davidson BR. A systematic review and meta-analysis of donor ischaemic preconditioning in liver transplantation. Transplant International. 2016;**29**(11):1147-1154. DOI: 10.1111/tri.12849

[67] Uemura T, Randall HB, Sanchez EQ, et al. Liver retransplantation for primary nonfunction: Analysis of a 20-year single-center experience. Liver Transplantation. 2007;**13**(2):227-233. DOI: 10.1002/lt.20992

[68] Coelho MPV, Afonso RC, Hidalgo R, et al. Results of retransplantation for

primary nonfunction in a single center. Transplantation Proceedings. 2011;**43**(1):174-176. DOI: 10.1016/j.transproceed.2010.12.003

[69] Yoo HY, Maheshwari A, Thuluvath PJ. Retransplantation of liver: Primary graft nonfunction and hepatitis C virus are associated with worse outcome. Liver Transplantation. 2003;**9**(9):897-904. DOI: 10.1053/jlts.2003.50176

[70] Stange B, Glanemann M, Nuessler NC, Settmacher U, Steinmüller T, Neuhaus P. Hepatic artery thrombosis after adult liver transplantation. Liver Transplantation. 2003;**9**(6):612-620. DOI: 10.1053/jlts.2003.50098

[71] Cavallari A, Vivarelli M, Bellusci R, Jovine E, Mazziotti A, Rossi C. Treatment of vascular complications following liver transplantation: Multidisciplinary approach. PubMed. 2001;**48**(37):179-183. Available from: https://pubmed.ncbi.nlm.nih.gov/11268960

[72] Karatzas T, Lykaki-Karatzas E, Webb M, et al. Vascular complications, treatment, and outcome following orthotopic liver transplantation. Transplantation Proceedings. 1997;**29**(7):2853-2855. DOI: 10.1016/s0041-1345(97)00706-9

[73] Cabezuelo JB, RamiRez P, Acosta F, et al. Prognostic factors of early acute renal failure in liver transplantation. Transplantation Proceedings. 2002;**34**(1):254-255. DOI: 10.1016/s0041-1345(01)02749-x

[74] Nüssler NC, Settmacher U, Haase R, Stange B, Heise M, Neuhaus P. Diagnosis and treatment of arterial steal syndromes in liver transplant recipients. Liver Transplantation. 2003;**9**(6):596-602. DOI: 10.1053/jlts.2003.50080

[75] Bekker JH, Ploem S, Jong DS. Early hepatic artery thrombosis after liver transplantation: A systematic review of the incidence, outcome and risk factors. American Journal of Transplantation. 2009;**9**(4):746-757. DOI: 10.1111/j.1600-6143.2008.02541.x

[76] Drazan KE, Shaked A, Olthoff KM, et al. Etiology and management of symptomatic adult hepatic artery thrombosis after orthotopic liver transplantation (OLT). PubMed. 1996;**62**(3):237-240. Available from: https://pubmed.ncbi.nlm.nih.gov/8607585

[77] Abbasoğlu O, Levy MF, Testa G, et al. Does intraoperative hepatic artery flow predict arterial complications after liver transplantation? Transplantation. 1998;**66**(5):598-601. DOI: 10.1097/00007890-199809150-00008

[78] Mourad MM, Liossis C, Gunson BK, et al. Etiology and management of hepatic artery thrombosis after adult liver transplantation. Liver Transplantation. 2014;**20**(6):713-723. DOI: 10.1002/lt.23874

[79] Pastacaldi S, Teixeira R, Montalto P, Rolles K, Burroughs AK. Hepatic artery thrombosis after orthotopic liver transplantation: A review of nonsurgical causes. Liver Transplantation. 2001;**7**(2):75-81. DOI: 10.1053/jlts.2001.22040

[80] Pinto LEV, Coelho G, Coutinho MMS, et al. Risk factors associated with hepatic artery thrombosis: Analysis of 1050 liver transplants. ABCD. 2020;**33**(4):75-81. DOI: 10.1590/0102-672020200004e1556

[81] El-Ella KA, Sebayel MA, Ramirez CB, Hussien RM. Outcome and risk factors of hepatic artery thrombosis after orthotopic liver transplantation in

adults. Transplantation Proceedings. 2001;**33**(5):2712-2713. DOI: 10.1016/s0041-1345(01)02157-1

[82] Rela M, Muiesan P, Bhatnagar V, et al. Hepatic artery thrombosis after liver transplantation IN children under 5 years of age. Transplantation. 1996;**61**(9):1355-1357. DOI: 10.1097/00007890-199605150-00012

[83] Mazzaferro V, Esquivel CO, Makowka L, et al. Factors responsible for hepatic artery thrombosis after pediatric liver transplantation. PubMed. 1989;**21**(1 Pt 2):2466-2467. Available from: https://pubmed.ncbi.nlm.nih.gov/2652807

[84] Rabkin JM, Orloff SL, Corless CL, et al. Hepatic allograft abscess with hepatic arterial thrombosis. American Journal of Surgery. 1998;**175**(5):354-359. DOI: 10.1016/S0002-9610(98)00051-8

[85] Crossin J, Muradali D, Wilson SR. US of liver transplants: Normal and abnormal. Radiographics. 2003;**23**(5):1093-1114. DOI: 10.1148/rg.235035031

[86] Oh C, Pelletier SJ, Sawyer RG, et al. Uni-and multi-variate analysis of risk factors for early and late hepatic artery thrombosis after liver transplantation. Transplantation. 2001;**71**(6):767-772. DOI: 10.1097/00007890-200103270-00014

[87] Kushner A. Virchow Triad. StatPearls - NCBI Bookshelf. Available from: https://www.ncbi.nlm.nih.gov/books/NBK539697/. Published December 10, 2022

[88] Duffy JP, Hong JC, Farmer DG, et al. Vascular complications of Orthotopic liver transplantation: Experience in more than 4,200 patients. Journal of the American College of Surgeons. 2009;**208**(5):896-903. DOI: 10.1016/j.jamcollsurg.2008.12.032

[89] Starzl TE, Porter KA, Putnam CW, et al. Orthotopic liver transplantation in ninety-three patients. Surgery, Gynecology & Obstetrics. 1976;**142**(4):487-505

[90] Mori K, Nagata I, Yamagata S, et al. The introduction of microvascular surgery to hepatic artery reconstruction in living-donor liver transplantation--its surgical advantages compared with conventional procedures. Transplantation. 1992;**54**(2):263-268. DOI: 10.1097/00007890-199208000-00014

[91] Zhao JC, Lu SC, Yan LN, et al. Incidence and treatment of hepatic artery complications after orthotopic liver transplantation. World Journal of Gastroenterology. 2003;**9**(12):2853-2855. DOI: 10.3748/wjg.v9.i12.2853

[92] Salvalaggio PR, Modanlou KA, Edwards E, Harper A, Abécassis M. Hepatic artery thrombosis after adult living donor liver transplantation: The effect of center volume. Transplantation. 2007;**84**(7):926-928. DOI: 10.1097/01.tp.0000281554.00247.92

[93] Piscaglia F, Vivarelli M, La Barba G, et al. Analysis of risk factors for early hepatic artery thrombosis after liver transplantation. Possible contribution of reperfusion in the early morning. Digestive and Liver Disease. 2007;**39**(1):52-59. DOI: 10.1016/j.dld.2006.08.004

[94] Silva MA, Jambulingam P, Gunson BK, et al. Hepatic artery thrombosis following orthotopic liver transplantation: A 10-year experience from a single Centre in the United Kingdom. Liver Transplantation. 2005;**12**(1):146-151. DOI: 10.1002/lt.20566

[95] Bilik R, Ra S, Phillips JO, Edwards V. Prevention of biliary cirrhosis following hepatic arterial thrombosis after liver

transplantation in children by using ursodeoxycholic acid. Journal of Pediatric Surgery. 1995;**30**(1):49-52. DOI: 10.1016/0022-3468(95)90608-8

[96] Nakazato P, Cox KL, Concepcion W, Berquist WE, Esquivel CO. Revascularization technique for reduced-size liver transplantation for infants weighing less than 10 kf. Journal of Pediatric Surgery. 1993;**28**(7):923-926. DOI: 10.1016/0022-3468(93)90698-k

[97] Atkison PR, Ross BC, Williams S, et al. Long-term results of pediatric liver transplantation in a combined pediatric and adult transplant program. CMAJ. 2002;**166**(13):1663-1671

[98] Tan KC, Yandza T, De Hemptinne B, Clapuyt P, Claus D, Otté JB. Hepatic artery thrombosis in pediatric liver transplantation. Journal of Pediatric Surgery. 1988;**23**(10):927-930. DOI: 10.1016/s0022-3468(88)80387-7

[99] Zuhair M, Smit GSA, Wallis G, et al. Estimation of the worldwide seroprevalence of cytomegalovirus: A systematic review and meta-analysis. Reviews in Medical Virology. 2019;**29**(3):e2034. DOI: 10.1002/rmv.2034

[100] Madalosso C, de Souza NF Jr, Ilstrup DM, Wiesner RH, Krom RA. Cytomegalovirus and its association with hepatic artery thrombosis after liver transplantation. Transplantation. 1998;**66**(3):294-297. DOI: 10.1097/00007890-199808150-00003

[101] Singhal A, Stokes K, Sebastián A, Wright HI, Kohli V. Endovascular treatment of hepatic artery thrombosis following liver transplantation. Transplant International. 2010;**23**(3):245-256. DOI: 10.1111/j.1432-2277.2009.01037.x

[102] Günşar F, Rolando N, Pastacaldi S, et al. Late hepatic artery thrombosis after orthotopic liver transplantation. Liver Transplantation. 2003;**9**(6):605-611. DOI: 10.1053/jlts.2003.50057

[103] Leonardi MI, Boin IFSF, Leonardi LS. Late hepatic artery thrombosis after liver transplantation: Clinical setting and risk factors. Transplantation Proceedings. 2004;**36**(4):967-969. DOI: 10.1016/j.transproceed.2004.03.121

[104] Levy AE, Larson A, Carithers RL, Perkins J. An analysis of late hepatic artery thrombosis after orthotopic liver transplant. Hepatology. 2000;**32**:214A-214A

[105] Margarit C, Hidalgo E, Lázaro JL, Murio E, Charco R, Balsells J. Biliary complications secondary to late hepatic artery thrombosis in adult liver transplant patients. Transplant International. 1998;**11**(Suppl. 1): S251-S254. DOI: 10.1007/s001470050472

[106] Sieders E, Peeters P, TenVergert EM, et al. Early vascular complications after pediatric liver transplantation. Liver Transplantation. 2000;**6**(3):326-332. DOI: 10.1053/lv.2000.6146

[107] Oh C, Sanfey H, Pelletier SJ, Sawyer RG, McCullough C, Pruett TL. Implication of advanced donor age on the outcome of liver transplantation. Clinical Transplantation. 2000;**14**(4):386-390. DOI: 10.1034/j.1399-0012.2000.14040502.x

[108] Pinna AD, Smith CV, Furukawa H, Starzl TE, Fung JJ. Urgent revascularization of liver allografts after early hepatic artery thrombosis1. Transplantation. 1996;**62**(11):1584-1587. DOI: 10.1097/00007890-199612150-00010

[109] Tzakis AG, Gordon RD, Shaw BW, Iwatsuki S, Starzl TE. Clinical presentation of hepatic artery thrombosis after liver transplantation IN the cyclosporine era. Transplantation. 1985;**40**(6):667-671. DOI: 10.1097/00007890-198512000-00019

[110] Heffron TG, Pillen T, Welch D, Smallwood G, Redd D, Romero R. Hepatic artery thrombosis in pediatric liver transplantation. Transplantation Proceedings. 2003;**35**(4):1447-1448. DOI: 10.1016/s0041-1345(03)00459-7

[111] Wozney P, Zajko AB, Bron KM, Point SW, Starzl TE. Vascular complications after liver transplantation: A 5-year experience. American Journal of Roentgenology. 1986;**147**(4):657-663. DOI: 10.2214/ajr.147.4.657

[112] García–Criado Á, Gilabert R, Nicolau C, et al. Early detection of hepatic artery thrombosis after liver transplantation by Doppler ultrasonography: Prognostic implications. Journal of Ultrasound in Medicine. 2001;**20**(1):51-58. DOI: 10.7863/jum.2001.20.1.51

[113] Vignali C, Bargellini I, Cioni R, et al. Diagnosis and treatment of hepatic artery stenosis after orthotopic liver transplantation. Transplantation Proceedings. 2004;**36**(9):2771-2773. DOI: 10.1016/j.transproceed.2004.10.028

[114] Brancatelli G, Katyal SL, Federle MP, Fontes P. Three-dimensional MULTISLICE helical computed tomography with the volume rendering technique IN the detection of vascular complications after liver transplantation. Transplantation. 2002;**73**(2):237-242. DOI:10.1097/00007890-200201270-00015

[115] De Gaetano AM, Cotroneo AR, Maresca G, et al. Color Doppler sonography in the diagnosis and monitoring of arterial complications after liver transplantation. Journal of Clinical Ultrasound. 2000;**28**(8):373-380. DOI: 10.1002/1097-0096(200010)28:8<373::aid-jcu1>3.0.co;2-b

[116] Langnas AN, Marujo W, Stratta RJ, Wood RP, Shaw BW Jr. Vascular complications after orthotopic liver transplantation. American Journal of Surgery. 1991;**161**(1):76-83. DOI: 10.1016/0002-9610(91)90364-j

[117] Saad WEA, Davies MG, Saad N, et al. Catheter thrombolysis of thrombosed hepatic arteries in liver transplant recipients: Predictors of success and role of thrombolysis. Vascular and Endovascular Surgery. 2007;**41**(1):19-26. DOI: 10.1177/1538574406296210

[118] Hidalgo EG, Abad J, Cantarero JM, et al. High-dose intra-arterial urokinase for the treatment of hepatic artery thrombosis in liver transplantation. Hepato-Gastroenterology. 1989;**36**(6):529-532

[119] Figueras J, Busquets J, Dominguez J, et al. Intra-arterial thrombolysis in the treatment of acute hepatic artery thrombosis after liver transplantation. Transplantation. 1995;**59**(9):1356-1357

[120] Yang Y, Li H, Fu BS, et al. Hepatic artery complications after orthotopic liver transplantation: Interventional treatment or retransplantation? Chinese Medical Journal. 2008;**121**(20):1997-2000

[121] Jain A, Reyes J, Kashyap R, et al. Long-term survival after liver transplantation in 4,000 consecutive patients at a single center. Annals of Surgery. 2000;**232**(4):490-500. DOI: 10.1097/00000658-200010000-00004

[122] Uzochukwu LN, Bluth EI, Smetherman DH, et al. Early postoperative hepatic sonography as a predictor of vascular and biliary complications in adult orthotopic liver transplant patients. American Journal of Roentgenology. 2005;**185**(6):1558-1570. DOI: 10.2214/ajr.04.1258

[123] Eurotransplant. Available from: https://www.eurotransplant.org/ [Accessed: August 2, 2023]

[124] Amitrano L, Guardascione MA, Brancaccio V, et al. Risk factors and clinical presentation of portal vein thrombosis in patients with liver cirrhosis. Journal of Hepatology. 2004;**40**(5):736-741. DOI: 10.1016/j.jhep.2004.01.001

[125] Manns MP. Liver cirrhosis, transplantation and organ shortage. Deutsches Arzteblatt International. Feb 2013;**110**(6):83-84. DOI: 10.3238/arztebl.2013.0083

[126] Ogren M, Bergqvist D, Björck M, Acosta S, Eriksson H, Sternby NH. Portal vein thrombosis: Prevalence, patient characteristics and lifetime risk: A population study based on 23,796 consecutive autopsies. World Journal of Gastroenterology. 2006;**12**(13):2115-2119. DOI: 10.3748/wjg.v12.i13.2115

[127] Van Thiel DH, Schade RR, Starzl TE, et al. Liver transplantation in adults. Hepatology. 2007;**2**(5):637S-640S. DOI: 10.1002/hep.1840020517

[128] Rugivarodom M, Charatcharoenwitthaya P. Nontumoral portal vein thrombosis: A challenging consequence of liver cirrhosis. Journal of Clinical and Translational Hepatology. 2020;**9**(1):1-13. DOI: 10.14218/jcth.2020.00067

[129] Stieber AC, Zetti G, Todo S, et al. The spectrum of portal vein thrombosis in liver transplantation. Annals of Surgery. 1991;**213**(3):199-206. DOI:10.1097/00000658-199103000-00003

[130] Nonami T, Yokoyama I, Iwatsuki S, Starzl TE. The incidence of portal vein thrombosis at liver transplantation. Hepatology. 1992;**16**(5):1195-1198

[131] Yerdel MA, Gunson BK, Mirza DF, et al. Portal vein thrombosis IN adults undergoing liver transplantation. Transplantation. 2000;**69**(9):1873-1881. DOI: 10.1097/00007890-200005150-00023

[132] Jamieson NV. Changing perspectives IN portal vein thrombosis and liver transplantation. Transplantation. 2000;**69**(9):1772-1774. DOI:10.1097/00007890-200005150-00006

[133] Charco R, Fuster J, Fondevila C, Ferrer J, Mans E, García-Valdecasas JC. Portal vein thrombosis in liver transplantation. Transplantation Proceedings. 2005;**37**(9):3904-3905. DOI: 10.1016/j.transproceed.2005.09.120

[134] Bauer JR, Johnson S, Durham JD, et al. The role of TIPS for portal vein patency in liver transplant patients with portal vein thrombosis. Liver Transplantation. 2006;**12**(10):1544-1551. DOI: 10.1002/lt.20869

[135] Ma J, Zhang Y, Luo J, Liu Q, Wang J, Qiu S. Rational classification of portal vein thrombosis and its clinical significance. PLoS One. 2014;**9**(11):e112501. DOI: 10.1371/journal.pone.0112501

[136] De Franchis R. Expanding consensus in portal hypertension. Journal of Hepatology. 2015;**63**(3):743-752. DOI: 10.1016/j.jhep.2015.05.022

[137] Sarin SK, Philips CA, Kamath PS, et al. Toward a comprehensive new

classification of portal vein thrombosis in patients with cirrhosis. Gastroenterology. 2016;**151**(4):574-577.e3. DOI: 10.1053/j.gastro.2016.08.033

[138] Ponziani FR, Zocco MA, Garcovich M, D'Aversa F, Roccarina D, Gasbarrini A. What we should know about portal vein thrombosis in cirrhotic patients: A changing perspective. World Journal of Gastroenterology. 2012;**18**(36):5014-5020. DOI: 10.3748/wjg.v18.i36.5014

[139] Denninger MH, Chaït Y, Casadevall N, et al. Cause of portal or hepatic venous thrombosis in adults: The role of multiple concurrent factors. Hepatology. 2000;**31**(3):587-591. DOI: 10.1002/hep.510310307

[140] Molmenti EP, Roodhouse TW, Molmenti H, et al. Thrombendvenectomy for organized portal vein thrombosis at the time of liver transplantation. Annals of Surgery. 2002;**235**(2):292-296. DOI:10.1097/00000658-200202000-00019

[141] Sogaard KK, Astrup LB, Vilstrup H, Gronbaek H. Portal vein thrombosis; risk factors, clinical presentation and treatment. BMC Gastroenterology. 2007;7:34. Published 2007 Aug 15. DOI: 10.1186/1471-230X-7-34

[142] Shukla A, Giri S. Portal vein thrombosis in cirrhosis. Journal of Clinical and Experimental Hepatology. 2022;**12**(3):965-979. DOI: 10.1016/j.jceh.2021.11.003

[143] Intagliata NM, Argo CK, Stine JG, et al. Concepts and controversies in haemostasis and thrombosis associated with liver disease: Proceedings of the 7th international coagulation in liver disease conference. Thrombosis and Haemostasis. 2018;**118**(8):1491-1506. DOI: 10.1055/s-0038-1666861

[144] Hoekstra J, Janssen HL. Vascular liver disorders (II): Portal vein thrombosis. The Netherlands Journal of Medicine. 2009;**67**(2):46-53

[145] Janssen HL, Wijnhoud A, Haagsma EB, et al. Extrahepatic portal vein thrombosis: Aetiology and determinants of survival. Gut. 2001;**49**(5):720-724. DOI: 10.1136/gut.49.5.720

[146] Englesbe MJ, Schaubel DE, Cai S, Guidinger MK, Merion RM. Portal vein thrombosis and liver transplant survival benefit. Liver Transplantation. 2010;**16**(8):999-1005. DOI: 10.1002/lt.22105

[147] Marini M, Castro-Lopez E, Manteiga DF, et al. Endovascular treatment of Spleno-mesenteric-portal vein thrombosis during Orthotopic liver transplant: 20 years later. Transplantation Proceedings. 2020;**52**(5):1459-1463. DOI: 10.1016/j.transproceed.2020.02.071

[148] Rajani R, Björnsson E, Bergquist A, et al. The epidemiology and clinical features of portal vein thrombosis: A multicentre study. Alimentary Pharmacology & Therapeutics. 2010;**32**(9):1154-1162. DOI: 10.1111/j.1365-2036.2010.04454.x

[149] Ponziani FR, Zocco MA, Campanale C, et al. Portal vein thrombosis: Insight into physiopathology, diagnosis, and treatment. World Journal of Gastroenterology. 2010;**16**(2):143-155. DOI: 10.3748/wjg.v16.i2.143

[150] Lebrec D, Bataille C, Bercoff E, Valla D. Hemodynamic changes in patients with portal venous obstruction. Hepatology. 1983;**3**(4):550-553. DOI: 10.1002/hep.1840030412

[151] Goulding C, Uttenthal B, Foroni L, et al. The JAK2(V617F) tyrosine kinase

mutation identifies clinically latent myeloproliferative disorders in patients presenting with hepatic or portal vein thrombosis. International Journal of Laboratory Hematology. 2008;**30**(5):415-419. DOI: 10.1111/j.1751-553X.2007.00973.x

[152] Zocco MA, Di Stasio E, De Cristofaro R, et al. Thrombotic risk factors in patients with liver cirrhosis: Correlation with MELD scoring system and portal vein thrombosis development. Journal of Hepatology. 2009;**51**(4):682-689. DOI: 10.1016/j.jhep.2009.03.013

[153] Francoz C, Valla D, Durand F. Portal vein thrombosis, cirrhosis, and liver transplantation. Journal of Hepatology. 2012;**57**(1):203-212. DOI: 10.1016/j.jhep.2011.12.034

[154] Maruyama H, Okugawa H, Takahashi M, Yokosuka O. De novo portal vein thrombosis in virus-related cirrhosis: Predictive factors and long-term outcomes. The American Journal of Gastroenterology. 2013;**108**(4):568-574. DOI: 10.1038/ajg.2012.452

[155] Kocher G, Himmelmann A. Portal vein thrombosis (PVT): A study of 20 non-cirrhotic cases. Swiss Medical Weekly. 2005;**135**(25-26):372-376. DOI: 10.4414/smw.2005.11035

[156] Ma SD, Wang J, Bezinover D, Kadry Z, Northup PG, Stine JG. Inherited thrombophilia and portal vein thrombosis in cirrhosis: A systematic review and meta-analysis. Research and Practice in Thrombosis and Haemostasis. 2019;**3**(4):658-667. Published 2019 Sep 10. DOI: 10.1002/rth2.12253

[157] Martinelli I, Primignani M, Aghemo A, et al. High levels of factor VIII and risk of extra-hepatic portal vein obstruction. Journal of Hepatology. 2009;**50**(5):916-922. DOI: 10.1016/j.jhep.2008.12.020

[158] Violi F, Ferro D, Saliola M, Quintarelli C, Alessandri C. Evaluation of D-dimer in patients with liver cirrhosis. Thrombosis and Haemostasis. 1989;**62**(4):1149-1150

[159] Tripodi A, Primignani M, Chantarangkul V, et al. An imbalance of pro- vs anti-coagulation factors in plasma from patients with cirrhosis. Gastroenterology. 2009;**137**(6):2105-2111. DOI: 10.1053/j.gastro.2009.08.045

[160] Stine JG, Argo CK, Pelletier SJ, Maluf DG, Caldwell SH, Northup PG. Advanced non-alcoholic steatohepatitis cirrhosis: A high-risk population for pre-liver transplant portal vein thrombosis. World Journal of Hepatology. 2017;**9**(3):139-146. DOI: 10.4254/wjh.v9.i3.139

[161] Stine JG, Shah NL, Argo CK, Pelletier SJ, Caldwell SH, Northup PG. Increased risk of portal vein thrombosis in patients with cirrhosis due to nonalcoholic steatohepatitis. Liver Transplantation. 2015;**21**(8):1016-1021. DOI: 10.1002/lt.24134

[162] Toth J, Barman P. Portal vein thrombosis: Before, during, and after liver transplant. Clinical Liver Disease. 2023;**22**(1):14-17. DOI: 10.1097/cld.0000000000000067

[163] Intagliata NM, Caldwell SH, Tripodi A. Diagnosis, development, and treatment of portal vein thrombosis in patients with and without cirrhosis. Gastroenterology. 2019;**156**:1582-1599.e1. DOI: 10.1053/j.gastro.2019.01.265

[164] Ak C, Adali G, Sayar S, et al. Portal vein thrombosis risk factors in liver transplant candidates. Hepatology Forum. 2022;**3**(3):88-92. Published 2022 Sep 23. DOI: 10.14744/hf.2022.2022.0005

[165] Gaballa D, Bezinover D, Kadry Z, et al. Development of a model to predict portal vein thrombosis in liver transplant candidates: The portal vein thrombosis risk index. Liver Transplantation. 2019;**25**(12):1747-1755. DOI: 10.1002/lt.25630

[166] Noureddin M, Vipani A, Bresee C, et al. NASH leading cause of liver transplant in women: Updated analysis of indications for liver transplant and ethnic and gender variances. The American Journal of Gastroenterology. 2018;**113**(11):1649-1659. DOI: 10.1038/s41395-018-0088-6

[167] Singal AK, Hasanin M, Kaif M, Wiesner R, Kuo YF. Nonalcoholic Steatohepatitis is the Most rapidly growing indication for simultaneous liver kidney transplantation in the United States. Transplantation. 2016;**100**(3):607-612. DOI: 10.1097/TP.0000000000000945

[168] Valla DC, Condat B. Portal vein thrombosis in adults: Pathophysiology, pathogenesis and management. Journal of Hepatology. 2000;**32**(5):865-871. DOI: 10.1016/s0168-8278(00)80259-7

[169] Englesbe M, Kubus J, Muhammad W, Sonnenday S, Welling T, Punch J, et al. Portal vein thrombosis and survival in patients with cirrhosis. Liver Transplantation. Jan 2010;**16**(1):83-90. DOI: 10.1002/lt.21941

[170] de Franchis R, Bosch J, Garcia-Tsao G, Reiberger T. Ripoll C; Baveno VII faculty. Baveno VII - renewing consensus in portal hypertension [published correction appears in J Hepatol. 2022 Apr 14;]. Journal of Hepatology. 2022;**76**(4):959-974. DOI: 10.1016/j.jhep.2021.12.022

[171] Tessler FN, Gehring BJ, Gomes AS, et al. Diagnosis of portal vein thrombosis: Value of color Doppler imaging. AJR. American Journal of Roentgenology. 1991;**157**(2):293-296. DOI: 10.2214/ajr.157.2.1853809

[172] Bach AM, Hann LE, Brown KT, et al. Portal vein evaluation with US: Comparison to angiography combined with CT arterial portography. Radiology. 1996;**201**(1):149-154. DOI: 10.1148/radiology.201.1.8816536

[173] Marshall M, Beese R, Muiesan P, Sarma D, O'Grady JP, Sidhu PS. Assessment of portal venous system patency in the liver transplant candidate: A prospective study comparing ultrasound, microbubble-enhanced colour Doppler ultrasound, with arteriography and surgery. Clinical Radiology. 2002;**57**(5):377-383. DOI: 10.1053/crad.2001.0839

[174] Hidajat N, Stobbe H, Griesshaber V, Félix R, Schröder R. Imaging and radiological interventions of portal vein thrombosis. Acta Radiologica. 2005;**46**(4):336-343. DOI: 10.1080/02841850510021157

[175] Loudin M, Ahn J. Portal vein thrombosis in cirrhosis. Journal of Clinical Gastroenterology. 2017;**51**(7):579-585. DOI: 10.1097/MCG.0000000000000834

[176] Mantaka A, Augoustaki A, Kouroumalis E, Samonakis D. Portal vein thrombosis in cirrhosis: Diagnosis, natural history, and therapeutic challenges. Annals of Gastroenterology. May-Jun 2018;**31**(3):315-329. DOI: 10.20524/aog.2018.0245

[177] Shah T, Semelka RC, Voultsinos V, et al. Accuracy of magnetic resonance imaging for preoperative detection of portal vein thrombosis in liver transplant candidates. Liver Transplantation. 2006;**12**(11):1682-1688. DOI: 10.1002/lt.20873

[178] Shaw BW Jr, Iwatsuki S, Bron K, Starzl TE. Portal vein grafts in hepatic transplantation. Surgery, Gynecology & Obstetrics. 1985;**161**(1):66-68

[179] Chen H, Liu L, Qi X, et al. Efficacy and safety of anticoagulation in more advanced portal vein thrombosis in patients with liver cirrhosis. European Journal of Gastroenterology & Hepatology. 2016;**28**(1):82-89. DOI: 10.1097/meg.0000000000000482

[180] Zanetto A, Rodriguez-Kastro KI, Germani G, et al. Mortality in liver transplant recipients with portal vein thrombosis - an updated meta-analysis. Transplant International. 2018;**31**(12):1318-1329. DOI: 10.1111/tri.13353

[181] Bhangui P, Lim C, Levesque É, et al. Novel classification of non-malignant portal vein thrombosis: A guide to surgical decision-making during liver transplantation. Journal of Hepatology. 2019;**71**(5):1038-1050. DOI: 10.1016/j.jhep.2019.08.012

[182] La Mura V, Braham S, Tosetti G, et al. Harmful and beneficial effects of anticoagulants in patients with cirrhosis and portal vein thrombosis. Clinical Gastroenterology and Hepatology. 2018;**16**(7):1146-1152.e4. DOI: 10.1016/j.cgh.2017.10.016

[183] Rodríguez–Castro KI, Vitale A, Fadin M, et al. A prediction model for successful anticoagulation in cirrhotic portal vein thrombosis. European Journal of Gastroenterology & Hepatology. 2019;**31**(1):34-42. DOI: 10.1097/meg.0000000000001237

[184] Loffredo L, Pastori D, Farcomeni A, Violi F. Effects of anticoagulants in patients with cirrhosis and portal vein thrombosis: A systematic review and meta-analysis. Gastroenterology. 2017;**153**(2):480-487.e1. DOI: 10.1053/j.gastro.2017.04.042

[185] Hanafy AS, Abd-Elsalam S, Dawoud MM. Randomized controlled trial of rivaroxaban versus warfarin in the management of acute non-neoplastic portal vein thrombosis. Vascular Pharmacology. 2019;**113**:86-91. DOI: 10.1016/j.vph.2018.05.002

[186] Hall TC, Garcea G, Metcalfe M, Bilku D, Dennison AR. Management of acute non-cirrhotic and non-malignant portal vein thrombosis: A systematic review. World Journal of Surgery. 2011;**35**(11):2510-2520. DOI: 10.1007/s00268-011-1198-0

[187] Cao G, Ko GY, Sung KB, Yoon HK, Gwon DI, Kim JH. Treatment of postoperative main portal vein and superior mesenteric vein thrombosis with balloon angioplasty and/or stent placement. Acta Radiologica. 2013;**54**(5):526-532. DOI: 10.1177/0284185113475917

[188] Walser E, McNees SW, Pena OD, et al. Portal venous thrombosis: Percutaneous therapy and outcome. Journal of Vascular and Interventional Radiology. 1998;**9**(1):119-127. DOI: 10.1016/s1051-0443(98)70493-2

[189] Luca A, Miraglia R, Caruso S, et al. Short- and long-term effects of the transjugular intrahepatic portosystemic shunt on portal vein thrombosis in patients with cirrhosis. Gut. 2011;**60**(6):846-852. DOI: 10.1136/gut.2010.228023

[190] Quencer K, Tadros A, Marashi KB, et al. Bleeding after percutaneous Transhepatic biliary drainage: Incidence, causes and treatments. Journal of Clinical Medicine. 2018;**7**(5):94. DOI: 10.3390/jcm7050094

[191] Kumar S, Sarr MG, Kamath PS. Mesenteric venous thrombosis. The New England Journal of Medicine. 2001;**345**(23):1683-1688. DOI: 10.1056/nejmra010076

[192] Joh JH, Kim D. i. Mesenteric and portal vein thrombosis: Treated with early initiation of anticoagulation. European Journal of Vascular and Endovascular Surgery. 2005;**29**(2):204-208. DOI: 10.1016/j.ejvs.2004.10.005

[193] Millis JM, Seaman D, Piper J, et al. Portal vein thrombosis and stenosis IN PEDIATRIC liver TRANSPLANTATION1. Transplantation. 1996;**62**(6):748-754. DOI: 10.1097/00007890-199609270-00008

[194] Tzakis AG, Kirkegaard P, Pinna AD, et al. Liver transplantation with cavoportal hemitransposition in the presence of diffuse portal vein thrombosis. Transplantation. 1998;**65**(5):619-624. DOI:10.1097/00007890-199803150-00004

[195] Yoshida EM, Erb SR, Morris DC, Wall W, Scudamore CH. Hepatic artery interruption followed by portal vein thrombosis in an adult liver transplant. Transplant International. 1994;**7**(6):434-437. DOI: 10.1007/bf00346038

[196] Miller C, Diago UT. The liver transplant operation. Clinical Liver Disease (Hoboken). 2013;**2**(4):192-196. Published 2013 Aug 19. DOI: 10.1002/cld.232

[197] Eghtesad B, Kadry Z, Fung J. Technical considerations in liver transplantation: What a hepatologist needs to know (and every surgeon should practice). Liver Transplantation. 2005;**11**(8):861-871. DOI: 10.1002/lt.20529

[198] Kruk E, Kalinowski P, Gibiński K, et al. Stapled anastomosis for side-to-side Cavo-Cavostomy in Orthotopic liver transplantation. Journal of Clinical Medicine. 2023;**12**(16):5289. Published 2023 Aug 14. DOI: 10.3390/jcm12165289

[199] Khorsandi SE, Athale A, Vilca-Melendez H, et al. Presentation, diagnosis, and management of early hepatic venous outflow complications in whole cadaveric liver transplant. Liver Transplantation. 2015;**21**(7):914-921. DOI: 10.1002/lt.24154

[200] Pfammatter T, Williams DM, Lane KL, Campbell DA Jr, Cho KJ. Suprahepatic caval anastomotic stenosis complicating orthotopic liver transplantation: Treatment with percutaneous transluminal angioplasty, Wallstent placement, or both. AJR. American Journal of Roentgenology. 1997;**168**(2):477-480. DOI: 10.2214/ajr.168.2.9016230

[201] Weeks SM, Gerber DA, Jaques PF, et al. Primary Gianturco stent placement for inferior vena cava abnormalities following liver transplantation. Journal of Vascular and Interventional Radiology. 2000;**11**(2 Pt 1):177-187. DOI: 10.1016/s1051-0443(07)61462-6

[202] Borsa JJ, Daly CP, Fontaine AB, et al. Treatment of inferior vena cava anastomotic stenoses with the Wallstent endoprosthesis after orthotopic liver transplantation. Journal of Vascular and Interventional Radiology. 1999;**10**(1):17-22. DOI: 10.1016/s1051-0443(99)70003-5

[203] Darcy MD. Management of venous outflow complications after liver transplantation. Techniques in Vascular and Interventional Radiology. 2007;**10**(3):240-245. DOI: 10.1053/j.tvir.2007.09.018

[204] Ko GY, Sung KB, Yoon HK, et al. Endovascular treatment of hepatic venous outflow obstruction after

living-donor liver transplantation. Journal of Vascular and Interventional Radiology. 2002;**13**(6):591-599. DOI: 10.1016/s1051-0443(07)61652-2

[205] Choi JW, Jae HJ, Kim HC, et al. Long-term outcome of endovascular intervention in hepatic venous outflow obstruction following pediatric liver transplantation. Liver Transplantation. 2015;**21**(9):1219-1226. DOI: 10.1002/lt.24215

[206] Emond JC, Heffron TG, Whitington PF, Broelsch CE. Reconstruction of the hepatic vein in reduced size hepatic transplantation. Surgery, Gynecology & Obstetrics. 1993;**176**(1):11-17

[207] Fujimoto M, Moriyasu F, Someda H, et al. Recovery of graft circulation following percutaneous transluminal angioplasty for stenotic venous complications in pediatric liver transplantation: Assessment with Doppler ultrasound. Transplant International. 1995;**8**(2):119-125. DOI: 10.1007/bf00344421

[208] Harihara Y, Makuuchi M, Takayama T, et al. Venoplasty of recipient hepatic veins in living-related liver transplantation. Transplantation Proceedings. Nov 1998;**30**(7):3205. DOI: 10.1016/s0041-1345(98)00995-6

[209] Ko GY, Sung KB, Yoon HK, et al. Early posttransplant hepatic venous outflow obstruction: Long-term efficacy of primary stent placement. Liver Transplantation. 2008;**14**(10):1505-1511. DOI: 10.1002/lt.21560

[210] Jang JY, Jeon UB, Park JH, et al. Efficacy and patency of primary stenting for hepatic venous outflow obstruction after living donor liver transplantation. Acta Radiologica. 2017;**58**(1):34-40

[211] Umehara M, Narumi S, Sugai M, et al. Hepatic venous outflow obstruction in living donor liver transplantation: Balloon angioplasty or stent placement? Transplantation Proceedings. 2012;**44**(3):769-771. DOI: 10.1016/j.transproceed.2012.01.048

[212] Quintela JM, Fernández C, Aguirrezabalaga J, et al. Early venous outflow obstruction after liver transplantation and treatment with Cavo-Cavostomy. Transplantation Proceedings. 2009;**41**(6):2450-2452. DOI: 10.1016/j.transproceed.2009.06.066

[213] Khan S, Silva MA, Tan YM, et al. Conventional versus piggyback technique of caval implantation; without extra-corporeal veno-venous bypass. A comparative study. Transplant International. 2006;**19**(10):795-801. DOI: 10.1111/j.1432-2277.2006.00331.x

[214] Kubo T, Shibata T, Itoh K, et al. Outcome of percutaneous Transhepatic Venoplasty for hepatic venous outflow obstruction after living donor liver transplantation. Radiology. 2006;**239**(1):285-290. DOI: 10.1148/radiol.2391050387

[215] Miraglia R, Maruzzelli L, Caruso S, et al. Interventional radiology procedures in Pediatric patients with complications after liver transplantation. Radiographics. 2009;**29**(2):567-584. DOI: 10.1148/rg.292085037

[216] Cheng Y, Chen CL, Huang T, et al. Angioplasty treatment of hepatic vein stenosis in pediatric liver transplants: Long-term results. Transplant International. 2005;**18**(5):556-561. DOI: 10.1111/j.1432-2277.2005.00088.x

[217] Yabuta M, Shibata T, Shibata T, et al. Long-term outcome of percutaneous interventions for hepatic venous outflow

obstruction after Pediatric living donor liver transplantation: Experience from a single institute. Journal of Vascular and Interventional Radiology. 2013;**24**(11):1673-1681. DOI: 10.1016/j.jvir.2013.07.010

[218] Cescon M, Grazi GL, Varotti G, et al. Venous outflow reconstructions with the piggyback technique in liver transplantation: A single-center experience of 431 cases. Transplant International. 2005;**18**(3):318-325. DOI: 10.1111/j.1432-2277.2004.00057.x

[219] Koç S, Akbulut S, Soyer V, et al. Hepatic venous outflow obstruction after living-donor liver transplant: Single center experience. Experimental and Clinical Transplantation. 2021;**19**(8):832-841. DOI: 10.6002/ect.2017.0045

[220] Köveker G, Viebahn R, Schott U, Judt-Stelzer G, Becker HD, Lauchart W. Hat die piggy-back Lebertransplantation einen nachteiligen Einfluss auf den venösen Abfluss?--Eine duplexsonographische Vergleichsstudie [does piggy-back liver transplantation have a detrimental effect on venous drainage?--A comparative duplex ultrasound study]. Langenbecks Archiv für Chirurgie. Supplement. Kongressband. 1996;**113**:402-404

[221] Arudchelvam J, Bartlett A, McCall J, Johnston P, Gane E, Munn S. Hepatic venous outflow obstruction in piggyback liver transplantation: Single Centre experience. ANZ Journal of Surgery. 2017;**87**(3):182-185. DOI: 10.1111/ans.13344

[222] Pandhi MB, Lipnik AJ, Niemeyer MM. Endovascular treatment of hepatic venous outflow obstruction after liver transplant. Digestive Disease Interventions. 2019;**03**(04):277-286. DOI: 10.1055/s-0039-3400494

[223] Navarro F, Le Moine MC, Fabre JM, et al. Specific vascular complications of orthotopic liver transplantation with preservation of the retrohepatic vena cava: Review of 1361 cases. Transplantation. 1999;**68**(5):646-650. DOI:10.1097/00007890-199909150-00009

[224] Morochnik S, Niemeyer MM, Lipnik AJ, Gaba RC. Immediate postoperative inferior vena cava stenting to improve hepatic venous outflow following orthotopic liver transplantation. Radiology Case Reports. 2020;**16**(2):224-229. Published 2020 Nov 28. DOI: 10.1016/j.radcr.2020.11.032

[225] Urahashi T, Mizuta K, Ihara Y, et al. Impact of post-transplant flow cytometric panel-reactive antibodies on late-onset hepatic venous outflow obstruction following pediatric living donor liver transplantation. Transplant International. 2014;**27**(3):322-329. DOI: 10.1111/tri.12255

[226] Sze DY, Semba CP, Razavi MK, Kee ST, Dake MD. Endovascular treatment of hepatic venous outflow obstruction after piggyback technique liver transplantation. Transplantation. 1999;**68**(3):446-449. DOI:10.1097/00007890-199908150-00018

[227] Ko GY, Sung KB, Gwon DI. The application of interventional radiology in living-donor liver transplantation. Korean Journal of Radiology. 2021;**22**(7):1110-1123. DOI: 10.3348/kjr.2020.0718

[228] Wang SL, Sze DY, Busque S, et al. Treatment of hepatic venous outflow obstruction after piggyback liver transplantation. Radiology. 2005;**236**(1):352-359. DOI: 10.1148/radiol.2361040327

[229] Shimizu Y, Yasargil MG, Smith RD. Thrombogenesis in experimental microvascular anastomosis. Journal of Microsurgery. 1979;**1**(1):39-49. DOI: 10.1002/micr.1920010105

[230] Pitchaimuthu M, Roll GR, Zia Z, et al. Long-term follow-up after endovascular treatment of hepatic venous outflow obstruction following liver transplantation. Transplant International. 2016;**29**(10):1106-1116. DOI: 10.1111/tri.12817

[231] Parrilla P, Sánchez-Bueno F, Figueras J, et al. Analysis of the complications of the piggy-back technique in 1112 liver transplants. Transplantation Proceedings. 1999;**31**(6):2388-2389. DOI: 10.1016/s0041-1345(99)00394-2

[232] Raby N, Karani J, Thomas S, O'Grady J, Williams R. Stenoses of vascular anastomoses after hepatic transplantation: Treatment with balloon angioplasty. AJR. American Journal of Roentgenology. 1991;**157**(1):167-171. DOI: 10.2214/ajr.157.1.1828649

[233] Lorenz JM, van Beek D, Funaki B, et al. Long-term outcomes of percutaneous venoplasty and Gianturco stent placement to treat obstruction of the inferior vena cava complicating liver transplantation. Cardiovascular and Interventional Radiology. 2014;**37**(1):114-124. DOI: 10.1007/s00270-013-0643-x

[234] Tasse J, Borge M, Pierce K, Brems J. Safe and effective treatment of early suprahepatic inferior vena caval outflow compromise following orthotopic liver transplantation using percutaneous transluminal angioplasty and stent placement. Angiology. 2011;**62**(1):46-48. DOI: 10.1177/0003319710369795

[235] Ferro C, Andorno E, Guastavino A, et al. Endovascular treatment with primary stenting of inferior cava vein torsion following orthotopic liver transplantation with modified piggyback technique. La Radiologia Medica. 2014;**119**(3):183-188. DOI: 10.1007/s11547-013-0325-4

[236] Ko EY, Kim TK, Kim PN, Kim AY, Ha HK, Lee MG. Hepatic vein stenosis after living donor liver transplantation: Evaluation with Doppler US. Radiology. 2003;**229**(3):806-810. DOI: 10.1148/radiol.2293020700

[237] Kumar G, Sharif K, Mayer D, et al. Hepatic venous outflow obstruction in paediatric liver transplantation. Pediatric Surgery International. 2010;**26**(4):423-425. DOI: 10.1007/s00383-010-2564-y

[238] Chong WK, Beland JC, Weeks SM. Sonographic evaluation of venous obstruction in liver transplants. American Journal of Roentgenology. 2007;**188**(6):W515-W521. DOI: 10.2214/ajr.06.1262

[239] Coulden R, Lomas DJ, Farman P, Britton PD. Doppler ultrasound of the hepatic veins: Normal appearances. Clinical Radiology. 1992;**45**(4):223-227. DOI: 10.1016/s0009-9260(05)80001-7

[240] Hwang HJ, Kim KW, Jeong WK, et al. Right hepatic vein stenosis at anastomosis in patients after living donor liver transplantation: Optimal Doppler US venous pulsatility index and CT criteria--receiver operating characteristic analysis. Radiology. 2009;**253**(2):543-551. DOI: 10.1148/radiol.2532081858

[241] Ripamonti R, Ferral H, Alonzo M, Patel NH. Transjugular intrahepatic portosystemic shunt-related complications and practical solutions. Seminars in Interventional Radiology. 2006;**23**(2):165-176. DOI: 10.1055/s-2006-941447

[242] Hausegger KA, Tauss J, Karaic K, Klein GE, Uggowitzer M. Use of the left internal jugular vein approach for transjugular portosystemic shunt. AJR. American Journal of Roentgenology. 1998;**171**(6):1637-1639. DOI: 10.2214/ajr.171.6.9843303

[243] Sze DY, Magsamen KE, Frisoli JK. Successful transfemoral creation of an intrahepatic portosystemic shunt with use of the Viatorr device. Journal of Vascular and Interventional Radiology. 2006;**17**(3):569-572. DOI: 10.1097/01.rvi.0000200054.73714.e1

[244] Quintini C, Miller CM, Hashimoto K, et al. Side-to-side cavocavostomy with an endovascular stapler: Rescue technique for severe hepatic vein and/or inferior vena cava outflow obstruction after liver transplantation using the piggyback technique. Liver Transplantation. 2009;**15**(1):49-53. DOI: 10.1002/lt.21667

[245] Kim KS, Lee JS, Choi GS, et al. Long-term outcomes after stent insertion in patients with early and late hepatic vein outflow obstruction after living donor liver transplantation. Annals of Surgical Treatment and Research. 2018;**95**(6):333-339. DOI: 10.4174/astr.2018.95.6.333

[246] Chu HH, Yi NJ, Kim HC, et al. Longterm outcomes of stent placement for hepatic venous outflow obstruction in adult liver transplantation recipients. Liver Transplantation. 2016;**22**(11):1554-1561. DOI: 10.1002/lt.24598

[247] Donaldson J, Obuchowski NA, Le RT, et al. Stenting for inferior vena cava stenosis after liver transplant. AJR. American Journal of Roentgenology. 2019;**213**(6):1381-1387. DOI: 10.2214/AJR.18.20915

[248] Lu KT, Cheng YF, Chen TY, et al. Efficiency of transluminal angioplasty of hepatic venous outflow obstruction in Pediatric liver transplantation. Transplantation Proceedings. 2018;**50**(9):2715-2717. DOI: 10.1016/j.transproceed.2018.04.022

[249] Duerig TW, Wholey MH. A comparisonofballoon-andself-expanding stents. Minimally Invasive Therapy & Allied Technologies. 2002;**11**(4):173-178. DOI: 10.1080/136457002760273386

[250] Scheinert D, Katsanos K, Zeller T, Koppensteiner R, Commeau P, Bosiers M, et al. A prospective randomized multicenter comparison of balloon angioplasty and infrapopliteal stenting with the sirolimus-eluting stent in patients with ischemic peripheral arterial disease: 1-year results from the ACHILLES trial. Journal of the American College of Cardiology. 2012;**60**(22):2290-2295. DOI: 10.1016/j.jacc.2012.08.989

[251] Settmacher U, Nüssler NC, Glanemann M, et al. Venous complications after orthotopic liver transplantation. Clinical Transplantation. 2000;**14**(3):235-241. DOI: 10.1034/j.1399-0012.2000.140309.x

Chapter 6

Liver Transplantation: An Updated Criteria Selection for HCC

Nam Hoang Duc

Abstract

In recent decades, hepatocellular carcinoma (HCC) has appeared as main indication (40–60%) of liver transplantation (LT) — one of the most effective treatments for the disease. Inclusion criteria play a pivot role in order to improve the survival outcomes, as well as to minimize the recurrent rate after LT. Indications for LT in HCC, previously based on static staging (principally tumor burden), turned to a more active process with supplementary tumor biology in response to local-regional treatment. This enables patients beyond the widely-accepted Milan criteria (MC) to access LT without discouraging outcomes. Though considered too strict, MC remains the cornerstone of inclusion criteria, while many others which increasing extend beyond Milan have been applied. The LT inclusion criteria for HCC vary according to each institution, region, and country (whether it performs deceased-donor LT or living donor LT) and adapted over time. These criteria in fact were the truly predictive models for the risk of recurrent, and therefore the survival outcome post-LT. This chapter focuses on recent inclusion criteria and liver allocation policy for LT in HCC throughout the world.

Keywords: liver transplantation, hepatocellular carcinoma, extended criteria, downstaging, bridging therapy, Milan criteria, UCSF criteria

1. Introduction

Hepatocellular carcinoma (HCC) is the sixth most frequent new tumor (>800,000 new cases annually worldwide), with a constantly poor long-term survival, resulting in atop 900,000 yearly deaths (the fourth most common cause of cancer-related mortality) [1]. In adults, HCC is the most frequent primary liver cancer [2]. A total of 70–90% of cases arise on a setting of chronic liver disease (mostly viral hepatitis and alcoholic liver disease) [3, 4]. The majority of HCC patients do not fit curative resection or LT when diagnosis [3].

Historically, HCC was associated with poor overall anticipation. LT was first recognized a prospective cure for the disease since the first case was performed in an adult HCC patient [5]. Thomas Starzl (USA, 1967) and Sir Roy Calne (Cambridge, England, 1968) were successful pioneers in human *orthotopic liver transplantation* (OLT) [6]. Early outcomes of LT in HCC were poor with high early HCC recurrence suggested that the recipients had advanced disease [4]. However, with the awareness that patients with smaller HCC nodules profit better from LT, particular criteria were proposed to help decision-making [7]. Mazzaferro et al. had milestone report that LT for HCC with certain limited criteria resulted in significant improval of *recurrence-free and overall survival at 4 years*, evidently specify the vitalness of patient selection [8].

The apparent attraction of LT against other modalities in HCC treatment is the ability to exclude the cancer and the primitive liver cirrhosis at the same time, thus reducing the risk of HCC recurrent on the remnant liver [5]. There is constantly considerable discrepancy worldwide between LT patients demand and liver graft supply. This inquire a reasonable selection of potential candidates in order to identify the suitable HCC patients anticipated to gain the superior benefit from the procedure while not disadvantaging non-cancer patients in the same waiting list for LT. HCC patients are aimed to achieve a long-term LT results equivalent to those transplanted for other etiology (e.g., liver cirrhosis, acute liver failure..). That is, conforming to the primary principle of transplant utility, LT should be limited in patients with expected 5-year survival over 70% and recurring <10–15% [9].

Allocation rules and priorities, as well as special treatment strategies in the waiting list, have, accordingly, been established and are still being refined to warrant fairness between patients listed for HCC and non-HCC causes [9].

2. Staging systems for hepatocellular carcinoma

The staging systems of HCC are clinically useful for management orientation; the decision-making should be individualized based on patient factors, tumor burden, pathological, hepatic function, etiology of liver disease, and biological tumor criteria [10]. There are also interactions between patient-tumor factors and treatment efficacy. No staging system is applicable to every HCC patient. Furthermore, most of the existed criteria composed of preoperative imaging studies for evaluation the tumor burden without the critical results from pathological analysis of explanted livers. Therefore, there was always disproportionate evaluation of the Milan criteria pre- and post-operatively [10].

At 2010 AHPBA (American Hepato-Pancreato-Biliary Association) HCC consensus conference, there existed 18 HCC staging or scoring systems in use worldwide [11]. *Modified TNM* classification of *UNOS (United Network for Organ Sharing)* (**Table 1**) together with *BCLC* (*Barcelona Clinic Liver Cancer*) (**Figure 1**) were among the most practical and universally used staging systems for HCC.

The TNM classification, though widely chosen for cancer staging, has inferior capability in anticipating long-term survival for HCC [14]. However, despite these facts, TNM is still a referred utility for pathological reports of explant liver. Limitations of this system are based on imaging and not actual histological findings, and imaging can underestimate tumor burden in stage II patients by 27 to 33%. Moreover, the severity of cirrhosis, critical for prognosis, is not part of TNM, and this system does not reflect survival after LT [15].

The superiority of BCLC staging system is its integration of liver function (Child-Pugh score), tumor characteristics (the number and size of nodules, vascular invasion, and extrahepatic spread), and performance status (**Figure 1**). It is the only system that recommends the best available management for each stage.

T1	**1 nodule <1.9 cm**
T2	1 nodule 2.0–5.0 cm; 2 or 3 nodules, all <3.0 cm
T3	1 nodule >5.0 cm; 2 or 3 nodules, at least one >3.0 cm
T4a	4 or more nodules, any size
T4b	T2,T3 or T4a plus gross intrahepatic portal or hepatic vein involvement as indicated by CT, MRI or ultrasound
N1	Regional (porta hepatis) nodes, involved
M1	Metastatic disease, including extrahepatic portal or hepatic vein involvement
Stage I	T1
Stage II	T2
Stage III	T3
Stage IVA1	T4a
Stage IVA2	T4b
Stage IVB	Any N1, any M1

T3 lesions that meet UCSF criteria (single lesion ≤6.5 cm or 2–3 lesions none >3 cm with a total tumor diameter of ≤8 cm) were classified as T3A. The other patients with T3 HCC exceeding these criteria were classified as T3B.

Table 1.
UNOS modified TNM staging classification for HCC [12].

3. Liver graft allocation policies, prioritization on the waiting list

With obvious chronic organ shortage worldwide and in the setting of death-donation liver transplant (DDLT), allocation policies have frequently refined during the last decades in order to diminish waiting-list mortality while assuring of best survival for HCC patients after LT.

3.1 Model of end-stage liver disease (MELD) score

The MELD score, an objective measure incorporating three quantitative values (serum creatinine, international normalized ratio [INR], and serum bilirubin), has proven to be a strong predictor of short-term mortality (3-month) in cirrhotic patients, including LT candidates [5]. It is then used to prioritize patients for DDLT; however, it underestimates the mortality risk in HCC patients *because their biologic MELD was usually low*. Accordingly, patients with HCC within Milan criteria (MC: single lesion ≤5 cm or up to 3 lesions ≤3 cm) were provided with additional MELD exception points starting in 2002 to balance their risk of tumor progression while awaiting LT compared to the 3-month liver-related mortality risk of non-HCC patients [16]. In 2002, the MELD score was proposed as the core system for organ allocation and implemented in the US first, then in most Western countries [5].

HCC patients are generally prioritized on the wait list for DDLT aiming to preclude tumor-advancement exceeding acceptable inclusion criteria, which sequentially leads to dropout from the wait list and deceased from cancer. In the US, despite the UNOS allocation system assigned some priority to HCC patients, dropout rates from tumor advancement were up to 25% at 1 year and 43% in 2 years' wait time by 2001 [15].

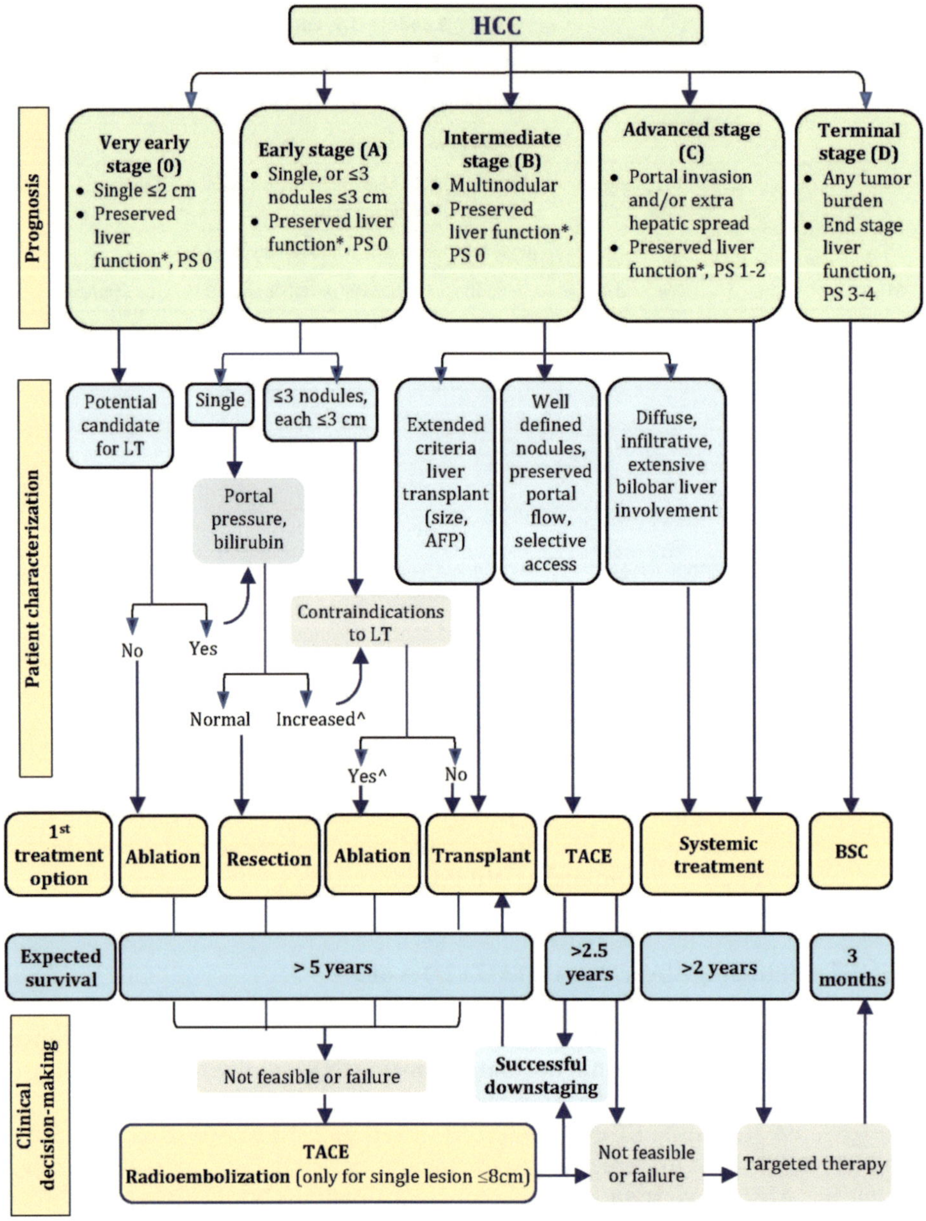

Figure 1.
*Modified BCLC staging and treatment strategy in 2022 [13]. * except for those with tumor burden acceptable for transplant. ^ resection may be considered for single peripheral HCC with adequate remnant liver volume AFP, alpha-fetoprotein; ALBI, albumin-bilirubin; BSC, best supportive care; ECOG-PS, eastern cooperative oncology group-performance status; LT, liver transplantation; MELD, model of end-stage liver disease; TACE, transarterial chemoembolization.*

In 2005, HCC patients within MC in the US irrespective of their biologic MELD score are listed with a score of 22 (**Table 2**). This resulted in a six-fold increase in LT for HCC and raising the concern non-HCC patients on the waiting list could be disbenefit by the allocation [17]. Ensuing data indicated extra-MELD points often over-emphasizing the risk of tumor advancement and consequent fatality.

Year	MELD Exception Points
2002	29 for T2 lesions
	24 for T1 lesions
2003	24 for T2 lesions
	20 for T1 lesions
2004	24 for T2 lesions
	No exception points for T1 lesions
2005	22 for T2 lesions
	No exception points for T1 lesions
2015	Natural MELD score at time of listing for T2 lesions
	28, after 6 months
	Maximum of 34 MELD exception points
Proposed changes	Requirement for locoregional therapy in patients with 2–3 cm HCC prior to applying for MELD exception points
	Allowing exception points for select patients with T3 HCC who are downstaged to T2

Table 2.
MELD exception points for patients with HCC [16].

Therefore, this MELD priority program has since been revised occasionally (**Table 2**) [16].

The "*cap and delay*" policy revision (2015) required a six-month interval before LT based on their assigned HCC-exception score to earn a MELD of 28 (**Table 2**). By extending the wait time, poor biologic tumors will be identified and vain LT may be preceded [18]. In the US in the 2 years just before and just after the policy change, HCC candidates had a 37% lower risk of wait-list death/dropout prepolicy and a comparable risk of death/drop-out postpolicy, establishing fairness between HCC and non-HCC candidates in wait list [19].

3.2 Organ procurement and transplantation network (OPTN)/united network for organ sharing (UNOS)

The traditional MELD score was not generated to anticipate the mortality risk in HCC patients with cirrhosis. Furthermore, some regions in the US, the wait time for OLT can be up to 24 months. Therefore, a supplemental system for prioritization was developed by the OPTN/UNOS that would provide these patients access to an allograft before their HCC advances beyond MC (**Table 3**). Notably, in 2016, the OPTN adopted a downstaging protocol for patients with HCC tumor burden beyond MC.

4. Current inclusion criteria for primary LT in HCC patients

The term liver transplant discussed here refers to primary LT. The LT inclusion criteria vary according to each institution, region, and country (whether it performs deceased-donor LT or Living Donor LT), and it may eventually change. These criteria in fact were the truly predictive models for the risk of recurrent, and therefore the survival

Selection for automatic exception score:
• AFP < 1000 ng/mL. If AFP ≥1000 ng/mL, it must fall below and remain <500 ng/mL after treatment.
AND
• Patients within Milan criteria: *1–2 tumors between 1 and 3 cm, or 1 tumor between 2 and 5 cm.*
OR
• Downstaged to Milan criteria by liver-directed therapy from initial downstaging criteria: one tumor between 5 and 8 cm, 2–3 none greater than 5 cm and sum <8 cm, 4–5 lesions all less than 3 cm and sum <8 cm.
Awarded MELD exception score:
• MMaT-3. After six-month wait, patients are awarded a fixed score of three points lower than median MELD at transplantation (MMaT-3) for patients transplanted within the area of distribution where the candidate is listed (distribution is a concentric circle model as of February 4, 2020.) *MMaT is recalculated every 6 months based on data of the 1 year before.*
Appeal to National Liver Review Board:
• Pathway for patients outside of above criteria or who may require a higher priority score. *Center must provide adequate medical justification for prioritization over other waiting candidates.*

Table 3.
US selection and allocation for HCC in 2020 [20].

outcome. They may comprise simply the radiologic factors, in combination with serologic factors, or recruiting pathological factors, responses to locoregional treatments.

4.1 Preliminary and Milan criteria

Initiative outcomes of OLT for HCC were dismal [21]. Early series of Thomas Starzl in the US and Roy Calne, Rudolf Pichlmayr, and Henri Bismuth in Europe encountered many HCC patients, including children; the longest survival was only 16 months and few survived more than 1 year [22]. Until the 1990s, poor outcomes in terms of overall recurrent rate (40% in 2 years with 81% mortality) and universal tumor recurrence of HCC brought the transplant community to abandon the procedure for primary liver tumors. HCC was proclaimed a relative contraindication to LT by the US Department of Health and Human Services in 1989 [20, 22].

Bismuth *et al.* were the first to recognize the efficacy and safety of LT in early-stage HCC. They determined definitive *Paul-Brousse Hospital Criteria "less than two tumor nodules and a maximum tumor diameter < 3 cm"* had lower recurrence after LT when compared to liver resection (**Table 4**) [42].

In 1996, Mazzaferro et al. published a benchmark study found that limited LT selection criteria (*single tumor ≤ 5 cm or up to three tumors, each ≤ 3 cm, without macrovascular invasion or extrahepatic spread*) led to similar outcomes when compared with non-HCC patients [8]. These Milan criteria (MC) were used by the United Network for Organ Sharing (UNOS) since 2002 to arrange the listing priority of HCC patients [21]. Consequently, MC has been included in the BCLC pretransplant staging, the American Association for the Study of Liver Diseases (AASLD), and the European Association for the Study of the Liver-European Organization for Research and Treatment of Cancer (EASL-EORTC) practice guidelines [43].

With extensive organ shortage worldwide, it is universally agreed to constrain LT to HCC cases within MC, particularly in the scene of DDLT. Although MC significantly contributed to LT clinical practice at first with prognostic potency and helped revival this demanding procedure; they are restricted, precluding certain candidates who can gain from LT [23]. In addition, these criteria are based only on the preoperative radiological aspect and lack of related factors that can impact HCC recurrence, especially tumor biology.

4.2 UCSF criteria

About 25% of recipients were eventually found exceeding the Milan criteria on the explant histology post-LT, regardless their 5-year survival was above 50% [43]. This led to initial expansion of the LT criteria for HCC with the *University of California San Francisco* (UCSF) criteria, which was less strictive (**Table 4**). With this modest extension of selection, the favorable improvement in survival of HCC with LT was still maintained.

4.3 Other extended criteria

Promising results of OLT relying on MC have encouraged inclusion more HCC candidates on the wait list. Extending the selection criteria might show excellent outcomes [9]. There have been more and more incorporated factors composing various inclusion criteria (**Figure 2**). However, MC remains the landmark for LTindications in HCC candidates and the basis for comparison with other proposed criteria [44].

Theoretically, at least three different schemes may be scheduled for the extension of the HCC criteria transplantation with deceased-donor grafts in Milan-out HCC patients, living donor LT for patients beyond MC, and successful downstaging to MC before LT in patients primarily Milan out [43]. Furthermore, practicing on expanded criteria emphasizes two crucial points that have to be defined a priori [22]:

a. What should be considered as an acceptable posttransplant outcome in HCC?

b. How much the extension of criteria disadvantages other non-HCC candidates?

4.3.1 Composite models combining tumor burden and biomarkers

AFP and descarboxy-prothrombin (DCP) were found to be relevant to the risk of recurrence at various cutoff values and independent from tumor burden (**Table 6**) [35]. In particular, pre-LT AFP and DCP levels, which reflect tumor differentiation as well as macro- and microvascular invasion [35], can be considered as a representative marker of cancer aggressiveness. Finally, increasing of AFP while on the waiting list negatively impacted outcome [33, 60].

- *"French AFP model"* or *AFP score* (**Table 4**): Based on above ground, a first composite model combining AFP values and tumor features at listing, followed by a quarterly reassessment during pre-LT follow-up was designed and prospectively validated in France [35]. This model was proved more accurate than MC to predict recurrence in patients meeting or not Milan criteria. This score has been validated in Italy [61], Spain [62], and Latin America [63]. The model was adopted by the French Organization for Organ Sharing (Agence de la Biomédecine) in 2013 as the official tool to select HCC patients, lead to a major change in LT indications policy there.

Authors, (Proposed year)	Criterion name, Country	Study period	No. of pts.#	Viral hepa-titis	Eligibility criteria	Survival within criteria*	
						Overall	RFS
Bismuth [24]	Paul-Brousse Hospital Criteria, France	1980–1991	60	—	1 or 2 nodules <3 cm (vs. ≥ 3 nodules, ≥ 3 cm)	83 vs.46% 3Y	83 vs.44% 3Y
Mazzaferro et al. [8]	Milan, Italy	1991–1994	48	HCV 70.8%, HBV 27.1%	Single tumor ≤5 cm; or 2–3 tumors ≤3 cm	85.0% at 4Y vs. 50.0%	92.0% at 4Y RFS vs. 59.0%
Yao et al. [14]	UCSF, USA	1998–2000	70	HCV 50.0%, HBV 18.6%	Single tumor ≤6.5 cm; or 2–3 tumors ≤4.5 cm and total diameter ≤ 8 cm	75.2% at 5Y	—
Herrero et al. [25]	CUN, Spain	1991–2000	47	HCV 60%	one ≤6 cm, or up to three ≤5 cm	79% 5Y	70% 5Y
Roayaie et al. [26]	Mount Sinai, USA	1991–1999	43	HCV 48.8%; HBV 23.2%	any number of lesions, each 5–7 cm in diameter	—	55% at 5Y vs. 34%
Kneteman et al. [27]	Edmonton, Canada	1996 ~ 2001	40	HCV 42.5%; HBV 30%	one <7,5 cm or any number < 5 cm in diameter	82.9% 4Y	76.8% 4Y
Onaca et al. [28]	Dallas, USA (Multi-center, 4 continents)	1992–2005	1206	HCV 48.9%; HBV 13.2%	One tumor ≤6 cm, or 2–4 tumors each ≤5 cm	55.1% 5Y	52.4% 5Y
Zheng et al. [29]	Hangzhou, China	2000–2007	195	HBV 100%	a. TTD ≤ 8 cm, or b. TTD >8 cm, and histopathologic grade I or II and preopeative AFP ≤ 400 ng/mL	46.2%	34.6%

Authors, (Proposed year)	Criterion name, Country	Study period	No. of pts.#	Viral hepa-titis	Eligibility criteria	Survival within criteria*	
						Overall	RFS
Silva et al. [30]	Valencia, Spain	1991–2006	257	HCV 61.4%; HCV+ alcohol 17.6%; HBV 6.7%	≤ three lesions, each ≤5 cm, TTD ≤ 10 cm	63% 5Y$	—
Mazzaferro et al. [31]	Up to Seven, (Multi-center)	2006–2007	283**	—	Sum of number of tumors and diameter (cm) of the largest tumor ≤7. No micro VI	71.2% at 5Y vs. 64.0%‡	9.1% at 5Y RR vs. 22.3%‡
Toso et al. [32]	TTV/AFP	2002–2008	5488	-	Total tumor volume ≤ 115 cm3 and AFP ≤ 400 ng/mL	<50% at 3Y (Patients not meeting)	—
Lai Q et al. [33]	AFP-TTD	Italy	158	HCV 58.2%, HBV 24.7%	TTD ≤ 8 cm and AFP ≤ 400 ng/mL	—	74.4%
DuBay et al. [34]	e-Toronto, Canada	1996–2008	294	HCV 52.0%, HBV 23.0%	• No tumor size or number restriction • No systemic symptoms and macro-VI • Not poorly differentiated cancer (if beyond MC)	79.0% at 5Y vs. 61.0%‡	76.0% at 5Y RFS vs. 58.0%‡
Duvoux et al. [35]	AFP, France	1988–2004	972	Hepa-titis 50.9%	Score ranged from 0 to 9 using AFP level, tumor diameter and number†	67.8% at 5Y vs. 47.5%	8.8% at 5Y RR vs. 50.6%
Grąt et al. [36]	Warsaw	1994–2012	121	HCV 63.6%, HBV 37.2%	beyond Milan, but within UCSF or up to 7 criteria with AFP < 100 ng/mL	—	100%
Mehta et al. [37]	RETREAT, USA	2000–2012	1061	HCV 62.8%, HBV 5.5%	Score ranged from 0 to 8 using AFP, mVI, tumor diameter and number of viable tumors of explant†	93.1% at 1Y; 77.0% at 5Y	2.9% at 5Y RR vs. 75.2% (score 0 vs. ≥5)

Authors, (Proposed year)	Criterion name, Country	Study period	No. of pts.#	Viral hepa-titis	Eligibility criteria	Survival within criteria*	
						Overall	RFS
Mehta et al. [38]	RETREAT, USA	2012–2014	3276	HCV 58.0%, HBV 18.3%	Score ranged from 0 to 8 using AFP, mVI, largest viable tumor plus number of viable tumors of explant†	93.1% at 1Y; 83.2% at 3Y	3Y RR of 1.6%, 8.4% and 29.0% for a score of 0, 3 and ≥ 5
Halazun et al. [39]	MORAL, USA	2001–2012	339	HCV 69.3%, HBV 15.3%	Pre-MORAL: NLR, maximum AFP and tumor size; post-MORAL: tumor grade, vascular invasion, tumor size and number on pathology†	—	Pre-MORAL: 98.6% at 5Y RFS in low risk
Mazzaferro et al. [40]	Metroticket 2.0, Italy. *Validated in China*	2000–2013	1359	HCV 56.9%, HBV 21.1%§	1. If AFP <200 ng/mL, sum of number and size ≤7 2. If 200 ≤ AFP <400 ng/mL, sum of number and size ≤5 3. If 400 ≤ AFP <1000 ng/mL, sum of number and size ≤4	79.7% at 5Y vs. 51.2%	89.6% at 5Y RFS vs. 46.8%
Goldberg et al. [41]	LiTES-HCC, USA	2002–2018	6502	HCV 43.0%	11 variables including liver related and non-related factors	86.3% at 5Y: (highest score)	—

All criteria require no macrovascular invasion.
HBV, HCV: hepatitis B, C virus; RFS, recurrence-free survival; RR, recurrence rate; VI, vascular invasion; TTV: Total Tumor Volume; TTD: Total Tumor Diameter; RETREAT, Risk Estimation of Tumor Recurrence After Transplant; mVI, microvascular invasion; NLR, neutrophil-to-lymphocyte ratio; LiTES-HCC, Liver Transplant Expected Survival-HCC. nY, n-years. #*Number of patients.*
**Survival of patients who met the criteria (compared with patients who did not meet the criteria).*
***Not clearly indicated DDLT or LDLT (mixed data).*
†*Detailed criteria for AFP, RETREAT, and MORAL (USA) scores are summarized in* **Table 5**.
‡*Survival and Recurrent Rate of the patients beyond Milan criteria but within vs. beyond Up to Seven criteria, each.*
$*Comparable to patients with tumors within MC.*
§*Training set (Italy): HCV 56.9%, HBV 21.1%; validation set (China): HCV 2.6%, HBV 96.2%.*

Table 4.
Criteria based on deceased-donor liver transplantation [2, 23].

		Point
AFP model	Total score > 2: 50.6% of 5-year recurrence rate	
	Tumor diameter:	
	≤3 cm	0
	3–6 cm	1
	>6 cm	4
	Number of tumors:	
	1–3	0
	≥4	2
	AFP (ng/mL):	
	≤ 100	0
	100–1000	2
	>1000	3
RETREAT	Score 5 or more: 75.2% of 5-year recurrence rate	
	AFP at LT (ng/mL):	
	0–20	0
	21–99	1
	100–999	2
	≥1000	3
	Microvascular invasion	
	Present	2
	Largest diameter + No. of viable tumors on explant	
	≤ 1 cm	0
	1.1–4.9 cm	1
	5–9.9 cm	2
	≥10 cm	3
MORAL (USA)	Pre-MORAL: Score > 10: 17.9% of 1-year RFS	
	Preoperative NLR, ≥5	6
	Maximum AFP, >200 ng/mL	4
	Largest tumor size, >3 cm	3
	Post-MORAL (pathology): Score > 10:	
	22.1% of 5-year RFS:	
	Grade 4 tumors, present	6
	Vascular invasion, present	2
	Largest size, >3 cm	3
	Tumor number, >3	2

RETREAT, Risk Estimation of Tumor Recurrence After Transplant; LT, liver transplantation; NLR, neutrophil-to-lymphocyte ratio; RFS, recurrence-free survival.

Table 5.
Specific criteria of AFP, RETREAT, and MORAL (USA) models [23].

- *Metroticket 2.0 (2018)* (**Table 4**): In general, the "*metro-ticket paradigm*" best demonstrates the present occasion; the further stretch we cover away from the standard criteria, the higher the price we will have to pay in terms of greater recurrence [40].

- *A-P Level* (Hokkaido Group, Japan, 2007) [10] and *A-P 200 criteria* (Pusan National University Yangsan Hospital, South Korea, 2016) [53]. Within MC, patients exceeding the *A-P 200 criteria* had significantly worse 3-year disease-free survival (DFS) compared to the ones within the *A-P 200* criteria (56% vs. 90.7%, P = .012). Patients exceeding Milan criteria, those within the *A-P 200 criteria* had a significantly higher 3-year DFS compared to the one exceeding the *A-P 200 criteria* (88.2% vs. 24.3%, P = .003). This *A-P 200 criteria* was also externally validated from another major LT center (Yonsei University College of Medicine, Korea) and observed similar results [53].

4.3.2 Tumor histology

The groups of Padova [64] and Toronto [65] found that in T3-HCC without poorly differentiated cancer on tumor biopsy before LT, and 5-year DFS rates >70% could be achieved. This again emphasizes the crucial importance of tumor biology in evaluation of the recurrent risk. The main drawback of this factor is the risk of tumor seeding along the needle tract and by *sample effect* (not properly manifest the precise tumor pathology) [66].

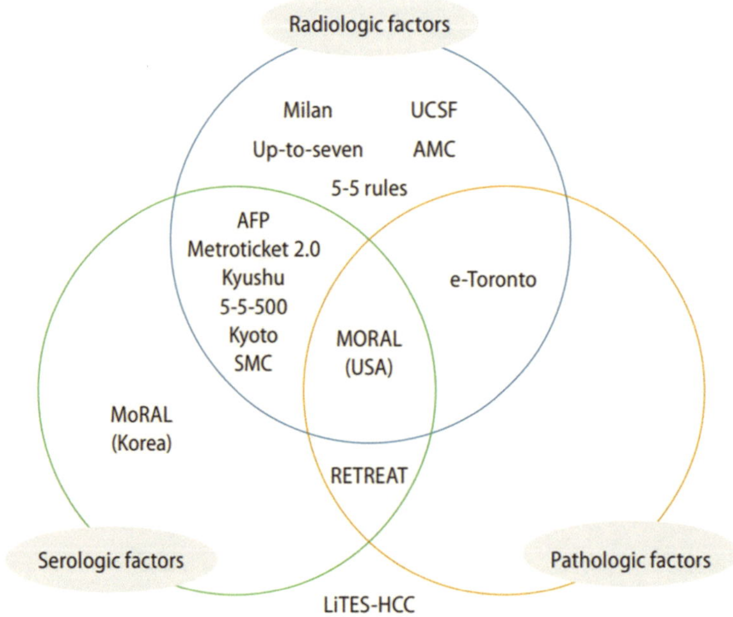

Figure 2.
Major prediction models based on recruited factors (reproduced with permission from [23]). AMC, Asan medical Center; SMC, Samsung medical Center; RETREAT, risk estimation of tumor recurrence after transplant; LiTES-HCC, liver transplant expected survival-hepatocellular carcinoma.

Authors, (Study period)	Criterion name (Country)	No. of pts.#	Viral hepatitis	Eligibility criteria	Survival within criteria*	
					Overall	RFS
Sugawara et al. [45] (1996–2005)	5–5 rule (Tokyo) (Japan)	78	HCV 62%	Number ≤ 5, Largest tumor ≤5 cm	—	94.0% at 3Y vs. 50%
Lee et al. [46] (1997–2004)	AMC (Korea)	221	HCV 62%, HBV 93.2%	Largest tumor ≤5 cm, number ≤ 6, no gross VI	76.3% at 5Y vs. 18.9%	—
Soejima et al. [47] (1996–2005)	Kyushu (Japan)	60	HCV 76.6%, HBV 15.0%	No limits for size and number of tumors, PIVKA-II ≤ 300mAU/mL	68.6% 3Y	*100% vs. 74% MC-out*
Chan et al. [48] (1996–2006)	University of Hong Kong (Hong Kong)	65	—	1 nodule of ≤6.5 cm	77.8% 3Y; 65.7% 5Y	—
Concejero, Chen et al. [49] (1999–2004)	Chang Gung Hospital (Taiwan)	35	All HCV+, HBV+ or combine	1 nodule ≤6.5 cm; or ≤ 3 tumors ≤4.5 cm	96% 3Y; 90% 5Y	—
Taketomi et al. [50] (1996–2007)	New Kyushu (Japan)	90	HCV 76.7%, HBV 13.3%	Tumor diameter ≤ 5 cm, or PIVKA-II ≤ 300mAU/mL	82.7% at 5Y	87.0% at 5Y
Ito, Takada, et al. [51] (1999–2006)	Kyoto *(10–5 rule)* (Japan)	125	HCV 53%, HBV 34%	≤ 10 tumors; all ≤5 cm and PIVKA-II ≤400mAU/mL	86.7% at 5-years vs. 34.4%	95.1% at 5-years vs. 60.5%
Furukawa et al. [52] 2007	A-P Level (*Hokkaido Group*) (Multi-center, Japan)	653	HCV 59%, HBV 30%	AFP ≤ 200 ng/ mL and PIVKA II ≤100 mAU/mL	—	At 5Y: 99.5% vs. 85.0% in MC-in; 84.3% vs. 45.0% in MC-out
Yang et al. [53]	A-P 200		—	AFP ≤ 200 ng/ mL and PIVKA II ≤200 mAU/mL	89.2% at 3Y vs. 80.0% ($p = .79$)	89.9% vs. 43.1% ($p < .001$)
Kaido, Mori et al. [54] (1999–2009**)	Kyoto (Japan)	176	HCV 71.6%, HBV 32.4%	≤ 10 tumors; all ≤5 cm and PIVKA-II ≤ 400mAU/mL	93% at 5Y vs. 25%, $p = .005$	90.0% at 5Y vs. 33.0%, $p = .011$

Authors, (Study period)	Criterion name (Country)	No. of pts.#	Viral hepatitis	Eligibility criteria	Survival within criteria*	
					Overall	RFS
Kim JM et al. [55] (2002–2008)	SMC (Korea)	180	HCV 6.7%, HBV 87.2%	Largest tumor ≤6 cm, number ≤ 7, and AFP ≤1000 ng/mL	—	90.0% at 5Y vs. 47.6%
Lee SD et al. [56] (2005–2013)	NCCK (*National Cancer Center Korea*) (Korea)	280	HBV 86.6%; HCV 5.5%; NANB 6.7%; HBV+ HCV 1.2%	negative PET/CT findings and total tumor size <10 cm	85.2%	84%
Lee JH et al. [57] (2001–2013)	MoRAL (Korea)	566	HCV 6.9%, HBV 87.8%	MoRAL score ≤ 314.8 Score calculation = $11 \times \sqrt{\text{PIVKA-II}} + 2 \times \sqrt{\text{AFP}}$	66.3% at 5Y†	82.6% at 5Y†
Lee EC et al. [58] (2005–2015)	GRWR	328	—	Beyond MC: SFSG (GRWR<0.8%)	—	*3Y: 49.3% vs. 68.3%; *5Y: 49.3% vs. 64.3%
Shimamura et al. [59] (1998–2009)	5-5-500 rule (Japan)	965	HCV 29.2%, HBV 60.3%	Tumor ≤5 cm, tumor number ≤ 5, AFP ≤ 500 ng/mL	75.8% at 5Y	73.2% at 5Y and a 19% increases number of eligible patients who are beyond MC

All criteria require neither extrahepatic metastasis nor macrovascular invasion.
NANB: non-A non-B hepatitis; PIVKA-II, prothrombin induced by vitamin K absence-II;
nY: n-years. MC-in: within MC; MC-out: exceeding of MC. SFSG: Small-for-Size Graft. #*Number of patients.*
**Survival of patients who met the criteria (compared with those who did not meet the criteria).*
†*Survival of the patients beyond MC but within MoRAL score ≤ 314.8.*

Table 6.
Criteria based on LDLT. (modified from [23]).

4.3.3 18 FDG pet CT

Certain retrospective studies from Germany and Korea have persistently shown that tumors with high FDG uptake have a significantly higher risk of recurrence compared to HCC with no or lower uptake because high SUV is significantly associated with poor differentiation and microvascular invasion (**Table 4**) [67]. In a recent Korean study, the combination of the positive FDG-PET study and AFP level > 200 ng/mL could better predict tumor recurrence after LDLT than MC. Moreover, LT in low SUV and low AFP pre-LT values was related with 80% 5-year survival rates, regardless of MC or tumor burden [56].

UCSF criteria combined with the FDG-PET condition can anticipate tumor recurrence after LDLT (tumor recurrence is earlier in cases with positive FDG-PET results) (a retrospective study in 2016 in Taiwan) [68].

This indicates that tumor biology might predict the recurrence risk better than tumor staging [9]. Impressively, 18 FDG PET-CT before LT can reveal undiagnosed extrahepatic metastases or additional intrahepatic tumors, enabling restaging of HCC in 10% of candidates [69].

4.3.4 Other recent prognostic variables and scores

Diverse parameters recently have been found valuable or validated as prognostic indicators or liberated risk factors for HCC recurrence after LT:

- *GRWR* (graft-to-recipient body weight ratio) (**Table 6**)

- Preoperative *CRP* (C-reactive protein): CRP >1 mg/dL was a separate risk factor for HCC recurrence with a 5-y recurrence rate of 27.4 vs. 16.4% (Meischl et al. 2019) [70].

- *ALBI* grade: It was measured employing pre-transplant serum albumin and bilirubin. Post-LT HCC recurrence rates were 10.5, 15.9, and 68.2% in ALBI grades 1, 2, and 3, correspondingly. Together with AFP and CRP, ALBI grades 1 or 2 were determined as an isolated predictor of RFS. ALBI grade 3 proved to be the strongest indicator of microvascular invasion (Kornberg et al. 2019) [71].

- The Hazard Associated with Liver Transplantation for Hepatocellular Carcinoma (*HALTHCC*) model determined as: (2.31*lin(AFP)) + (1.33*tumor burden score) + (0.25*MELD-Na) – (5.57*Asia). This score predicted overall survival, recurrence rate, and vascular invasion, poorly differentiated components on explant pathology (Firl et al., 2019) [72].

LDLT has been applied extensively in Asia as aforementioned, and many major centers soon recognized the crucial roles of AFP and PIVKA-II as the main recurrent predictors of HCC post-LT. Tumor burden had also been significantly expanded (**Table 6**).

5. Management in the waiting list: Downstaging or bridging therapy

Organ shortage is one of the main drawbacks of OLT. With biologic MELD score generally low, HCC candidates for LT are often struggled with prolonged wait times for DDLT. This may result in tumor growth exceeding the MC while in the wait list.

Median wait time of a HCC candidate ranges from 3 to 15 months [9]. Subsequently, whereas drop-out rate from LT wait list is around 15–30% due to HCC advancement, downstaging, and bridging management should be provided in patients with an estimating wait time for LT over 6 months [73]. That is, once they are registered for LT, and wait time of longer than 6 months is anticipated, locoregional therapies (LRT) for HCC will be carried out in order to satisfy certain criteria for OLT (*downstaging strategy*) or to assure the remnant tumors still stay within MC (*bridging therapy)* [2, 17].

LT after successful downstaging should aim to gain a 5-year survival equivalent to that of HCC recipients undergone LT without necessity of downstaging [44].

Bridging therapy approaches should be determined by pluridisciplinary board meetings, *transarterial chemoembolization* (TACE) was the most common modality. Approximately 25% of LT applicants are suitable to bridging management (probable curing), such as thermoablation or liver resection. Emergent approaches for instance *radioembolization* (TARE), *stereotactic external beam radiotherapy* (SBRT), and still *tyrosinekinase inhibitors* (sorafenib, levantinib...) were less recommended. Tiny central tumors in compensated liver cirrhosis were more suitable to treat with RFA, whereas larger tumors but sustained liver function are treated with TACE/TARE. In decompensated liver cirrhosis and larger tumor size, external radiotherapy may be recommended without increasing the risk of furthermore decline of liver function [74].

Registered Criteria:
HCC out of Milan criteria but fulfilled one of the following: 1. Single lesion 5.1–8 cm 2. 2–3 lesions each ≤5 cm with total tumor diameter ≤ 8 cm 3. 4–5 lesions each ≤3 cm with total tumor diameter ≤ 8 cm Without vascular invasion or extrahepatic spread on cross-sectional imaging
criteria for successful downstaging:
Residual tumor burden fulfilled Milan criteria (1 lesion ≤5 cm, 2–3 lesions ≤3 cm): a. Only effective tumor(s) are counted; tumor size estimations should not comprise necrotic regions after treatment. b. If more than one area of remnant tumor enhancement, then the size of the entire lesion should be calculated toward the overall tumor burden
Criteria for downstaging failure and dropout of wait list:
1. Advancement of tumor(s) exceeding registration/qualification criteria for downstaging (described above) 2. Tumor macroscopic vascular invasion on cross-sectional imaging 3. Lymph node or extrahepatic metastasis 4. Tumor progress in the type of infiltration 5. In UNOS present principle, once AFP ≥ 1000 ng/mL, LT is not attempted until this marker drops below 500 ng/mL after LRT
Schedule of LT in regard to downstaging:
1. Minimal monitoring interval is supposed to be at least 3 months of tumor steadiness from accomplished downstaging to LT. 2. In UNOS present principle, candidates must reside inner of Milan criteria for 6 months after accomplished downstaging to receive MELD exception points.

Table 7.
UNOS downstaging criteria [77].

Authors; Study Period	Criterion, country	No. of patients (drop-out rate)	Viral hepatitis	Criteria	
				DS inclusion	Transplantation factor
Lai et al. [33] 1999–2010	No-named, Europe (6 centers)	422	HCV 45.5% HBV 15.9%	Exceeding MC	After downstaging, no risk of 1. AFP slope > 15 mg/mL/month; or 2. disease advancement mRECIST
Yao et al. [32] 2002–2012	UCSF downstaging, USA	DS: 118 (34.7%) vs. LT only: 488	HCV 56% HBV 27%	Single lesion: >5 cm and ≤ 8 cm; 2–3 lesions: at least one lesion >3 cm and ≤ 5 cm, total diameter ≤ 8 cm; 4–5 lesions: each ≤3 cm, total diameter ≤ 8 cm	DDLT: within UNOS criteria T2 LDLT: within UCSF criteria
Lai et al. [79] 2000–2014	TRAIN, Italy, Belgium	289	HCV 47.1% HBV 18.0%	Exceeding MC	TRAIN score ≤ 1.0 recommended Train score = 0.988 (if mRECIST-PD) + 0.838 (if AFPslope 15.0 ng/mL/month) + 0.452 (if NLR ≥5.0) − 0.03 × WT (month)
Mazzaferro et al. [80] 2011–2015	XXL criteria, Italy	DS: 74 (39.1%)	HCV 62.2% HBV 15.6%	Exceeding MC, age 18–65 years, Child-Pugh A–B (7), no MacroVI or extrahepatic spread	Complete response or partial response

DS, downstaging; HCV, hepatitis C virus; HBV, hepatitis B virus; RECIST, Response Evaluation Criteria in Solid Tumors; TRAIN, time-radiological-response-alpha-fetoprotein-inflammation; PD, progressive disease; NLR, neutrophil-to-lymphocyte ratio; WT, waiting time; VI, vascular invasion.

Table 8.
Downstaging procedures before liver transplantation [23].

Results of bridging management, evaluated with tumor size and AFP levels, should be carefully and routinely rechecked until LT. Tumor advancement [75] and AFP rising [60] during bridging therapies anticipate recurrence post-LT. Patients advancing beyond LT criteria should be resigned from the wait list. Conversely, candidates initially out of inclusion criteria can be effectively down-staged and, thereafter, registered for LT [76]. Downstaging within Milan (T2) criteria is achievable in 40% of those cases. The risk of HCC recurrence after a downstaging procedure is about 15% but still consistent with admissible 5-year survival rates roughly 70% [9].

To standardize downstaging criteria in the USA, UNOS/OPTN adopted the UNOS/Region 5 down-staging protocol (UNOS-DS; **Table** 7) in 2017, candidates who successfully downstaged to within MC qualified to obtain automatic MELD exception after the mandatory six-month waiting period [77].

Authors, (year report)	Criteria to enter DS	DS model (Nb of pts.)	Time stable prior to LT	DS success rate	LT criteria	LT rate	Post-LT survival, time, and rate (%)	r-HCC
Roayaie et al. [26]	Mount Sinai protocol: unresectable HCC > 5 cm	TACE (43)	—	—	—	53.75%	5 yr. OS 44% 5 yr. DFS 48% 5 yr. DFS: tumors 5–7 cm (55%) vs. tumor >7 cm (34%)	40%
Graziadei et al. [82]	Beyond Milan, no upper limit, no vascular invasion, no extrahepatic metastasis	TACE	No limit	73%	50% of tumor size	66.6%	4 yr. OS 41%; 5 yr. I-to-T 31%	30%
Otto et al. [83]	Beyond Milan, no extrahepatic metastasis	TACE (62)	No limit	55%	30% decrease in the diameter of 5 target lesions	—	74.5% at 5 yr.	—
Millonig et al. [84]	UCSF				RECIST	84.8%	5 yr. CR 66.6%; PR 63.7%; NR 25%	25%
Ravaioli et al. [78]	Bologna Criteria Beyond Milan: 1. 1 lesion ≤6 cm, 2. 2 lesions ≤5 cm, 3. 3–5 lesions ≤4 cm and TTD ≤ 12 cm	TACE, RFA, PEI and/or resection (48)	At least 3 months (mean: 6 months)	90%	To Milan: 72.9%	66.7%	3 yr. DFS 71% 3 yr. I-to-T 56.3%	15% at 3 year
Chapman et al. [85]	Beyond Milan, no lobar major vessel involvement or metastasis	TACE (76)	usually at least 4 months (mean: 6 months)	23.7%	To Milan	33.1%	100% at 3 yr. 50% at 5 yr	—

Authors, (year report)	Criteria to enter DS	DS model (Nb of pts.)	Time stable prior to LT	DS success rate	LT criteria	LT rate	Post-LT survival, time, and rate (%)	r-HCC
Lewandowski et al. [86]	T3	* TACE (43) * TARE-Y90 (43)	No limit	* 31% * 58%	To Milan	—	*1 yr. DFS 73% 3 yr. I-to-T 19% *1 yr. DFS 89% 3 yr. I-to-T 59%	—
De Luna et al. [87]	Beyond Milan	TACI (27)	no limit (mean: 11 months)	63%	To Milan	—	3 yr. OS 78.8% 3 yr. I-to-T 84%	—
Jang et al. [88]	Beyond Milan, no lobar major vessel involvement or metastasis	TACE (386)	no limit (median: 2 months)	41.5%	To Milan	—	5 yr. DFS 66.3% 5 yr. I-to-T 25%	—
Yao et al. [76]	UCSF downstaging Beyond Milan: • single tumor≤8 cm, • 2–3 tumors (at least one >3 and ≤ 5 cm, TTD ≤ 8 cm), • 4–5 tumors each ≤3 cm and TTD ≤ 8 cm				To Milan: 65.3%	54.2	5 yr. OS 77.8% 5 yr. I-to-T 56.1%	7.8

DS: Downstaging; Nb of pts.: number of patients; RFA: radio-frequency ablation; TACE: transarterial chemo-embolization; TACI: transcatheter arterial chemoinfusion, TARE-Y90: transarterial radioembolization with Yttrium-90 microspheres;; TTD: Total tumor diameter; yr.: year; OS: Overall survival; DFS: Disease-free survival; I-to-T: Intention to treat; rHCC: HCC recurrent.

Table 9.
Certain reports on downstaging before LT. (modified from [23]).

Authors, (year report)	Patient number	Findings
Pommergaard et al. [89]	4978 LRT of 23,124 LT recipients with HCC	LRT corresponded with better OS (HR 0.84 [0.73–0.96]) and HCC-specific survival (HR 0.76 [0.59–0.98]) post-LT. RFA was highly effective for OS and HCC-specific survival after LT.
Ogawa et al. [90]	223 LT recipients with HCC	In regard to number of pretreatments, recurrent rate was considerably greater in the ≥5 pretreatments group than the 0 group. Nevertheless, those fulfilled Kyoto criteria. no considerable differences in recurrent rates between groups.
Mehta et al. [91]	407 HCC recipients with AFP > 1000 ng/mL at LT wait list	5-y OS: AFP >1000 at LT; 48.8%, AFP to 101–499; 67.0%, AFP to <100; 88.4% 5-y HCC recurrent probability: AFP >1000; 35.0%, AFP to 101–499; 13.3%, AFP to <100; 7.2% In multivariate analysis, AFP decrease to 101–499 was related with a > 2-fold decrease in posttransplant mortality (*P* = .01) and a nearly 3-fold decrease in HCC recurrence (*P* = .02) [91]
Sinha et al. [92]	UNOS database of 3819 HCC LT; constantly fulfilled Milan (n = 3276), UNOS-DS (n = 422), and AC-DS (n = 121)	On explant, vascular invasion presented in 23.7% of AC-DS versus 16.9% of UNOS-DS and 14.4% of Milan (*P* = .002). Within DS groups, risk of post-LT death was higher in SWR or MWR and with AFP >100 ng/mL at LT. The 3-y HCC recurrence probability was 6.9% for Milan, 12.8% for UNOS-DS, and 16.7% for AC-DS (*P* < .001). In DS groups, AFP >100 was the only separate predictor of HCC recurrence. [92]
Vutien et al. [93]	16,558 HCC patients underwent LT in SRTR data	HCC burden measured at three points on the initial wait list (I), maximum (M) total tumor diameter, and last (L) exception petition. Classification: (A) < Milan (B) Milan (C) > Milan to UCSF (D) > UCSF. 1233 (7%) had any post-LT rHCC. rHCC rates were higher in RH-IML group CCC (15%) and DDD (18%). Low recurrence rates: M and L tumor burden did not exceed Milan (class A or B), effective downstaging when L was A(<Milan), and M tumor burden did not exceed I
DiNorcia et al. [94]	4109 patients for validation between 2015 and 2017	compared to patients without cPR, cPR patients were younger; had lower MELD scores, AFP levels, and NLR; were more probable having tumors within MC and fewer LRT treatments; and had significantly lower 1-, 3-, and 5-y incidence of post-LT recurrence (1.3, 3.5, and 5.2% vs. 6.2, 13.5, and 16.4%; *P* < .001) and higher general survival (92, 84, and 75 vs. 90, 78, and 68%; *P* < .001). Multivariable predictors of cPR included age, sex, liver disease diagnosis, MELD, AFP, NLR, radiographic Milan status, and number of LRT treatments.

Abbreviations: AC-DS, all-comers downstaging; SWR: short wait regions; MWR: mild wait regions; cPR, complete pathological response; HR, hazard ratio; Kyoto criteria, tumor number ≤ 10, maximal diameter of each tumor ≤5 cm, and DCP levels of ≤400 mAU/mL; OS, overall survival; rHCC, recurrent HCC; UCSF criteria, 1 tumor >5 cm and up to 6.5 cm or 3 tumors each up to 4.5 cm; UNOS-DS, (one lesion >5 cm and ≤ 8 cm; 2–3 lesions each ≤5 cm; or 4–5 lesions each ≤3 cm with total tumor diameter ≤ 8 cm) downstaging [70].

Table 10.
Essential updates of downstaging HCC before liver transplantation [70].

The inclusion criteria, aim, and protocols of downstaging still differ between centers; however, the general and initial aim is fulfilled Milan criteria (MC-IN) [78]. The European Association for the Study of the Liver (EASL) proposes LT only for MC-IN candidates after downstaging. The UCSF group introduced their *downstaging protocol* and defined the "*success of downstaging*" criteria, allowing more candidates to profit from LRT before LT (**Table 8**) [23]. Recent AASLD guidelines recommended that candidates beyond MC (T3) can be registered for LT after effective downstaging into MC [81]. Recent prospective studies and essential updates of HCC-downstaging before LT were summarized in the **Tables 9** and **10**.

6. LDLT for HCC

Due to important shortage of donated organs, with additional challenge of equal allocation of available organs among cancer *vs.* non-cancer recipients, certain surgical strategies have been established. All these approaches contribute the so-called "marginal graft" (also specified as "extended criteria livers"). Marginal grafts explication incorporates: (i) *Living donor right lobe graft*, *cadaveric liver division* (split the whole liver from cadaveric donors to two recipients of different size), (ii) *serious hepato-steatosis* (i.e., macrovesicular >60%), and (iii) organs harvested from *heartbeat brain death (DBD donors)* and even from *non-heartbeat* (circulation-death - *DCD donors*) [6].

LDLT has flourished in eastern countries (especially Japan, South Korea, Taiwan..) due to significant cadaveric organ shortage. Though DDLT has recently accounted above 90% of LT in the Western world, LDLT is predominant in many Asian centers [5]. LDLT has also been utilized in Western countries (with well-established programs for DBD or DCD programs), because of persistent organ shortage, prolong wait times related with wait-list mortality, disqualified because of health problems, or tumor advancement exceeding eligible criteria [44].

Concern still remains whether LDLT for HCC attains equivalent outcomes with DDLT, especially in MC-out candidates. Also, tumor recurrent rate has been reported higher in LDLT than DDLT [95]. However, at least two systematic reviews [96, 97] found no evidence to demonstrate this trend. Theoretically, several hypotheses were made on greater recurrent rates in LDLT: (1) Because of relative brief wait time for LDLT candidates, advancement of aggressive HCC biology could be neglected; while they might fall out from the wait list in DDLT setting and could not access to LT. This is the renown "*fast-track effect.*" (2) Growth factors and cytokines produced during speedy regeneration of the partial grafts might contribute to tumor advancement and recurrence. Nevertheless, there is lack of prospective study on this issue previously [98].

LDLT is more favorable than DDLT in reduced wait time, superior quality graft with better liver function, reduced ischemic time, and pretransplant treatment optimization for HCC that might contribute to enhanced survival of recipients with LDLT [98]. In the setting of LDLT, organs are donated as private gifts and not the public resources to allocate. Accordingly, many Asian centers have adopted their own extended inclusion criteria for LDLT for HCC with equivalent long-standing consequences based on HCC tumor burden [99].

7. Re-transplantation for HCC patient: The indications, considerations

HCC recurrence after LT mainly affects the liver graft itself and extrahepatic metastasis, commonly lungs, bone, and lymph nodes [9].

Retransplantation (ReLT) remains the only life-rescuing alternative in case of graft failure. Anyway, in spite of current ameliorations, its survival result was obviously unsatisfactory in comparison with primary LT [100]. According to European Liver Transplant Registry (ELTR) study (1998–2009), HCC recurrence was the indication in only 11% of cases [101].

Utilization of deceased-donor organs is usually justified for graft failure after LDLT. ReLT due to graft failure after LDLT was uncommon, but results are still favorable when required. The panel allowed reLT in LDLT recipients who initially fulfilled accepted criteria for LT. However, based on utility, justice, and equity, they would not support reLT for those previously exceeding these criteria since these patients would have been disqualified for DDLT in that priority. Acceptance reLT for this kind of patients would interfere others on the DDLT wait list and raise an "*ethical dilemma*" [44, 52]. It is the enigma of the "*200% mortality rate*" not only this recipient who ultimately diseases from cancer recurrence after transplantation but also other potential candidates, who rather obtain that graft but then advance to liver failure, disqualified from the list or died while waiting [22, 100].

ReLT recipients frequently present higher mean MELD than those of primary LT [102]. The MELD threshold for *survival benefit* (SB) from ReLT is 21, which is higher than the MELD threshold of 15 for primary LT. The mortality risk or graft failure after ReLT is 3.5–8.3 times higher than those without ReLT for recurrent candidates with MELD <21 [103].

Whereas there is no current agreement, 1-year predictable survival of at least 50% should be considered as effective reLT [100]. Several models for risk-predictor have been suggested so far to help avoid ineffective reLT and to facilitate the best judgment in allocation of organs in short supply. Rosen proposed the most frequently employed risk score for reLT in 1999 and validated in 2003 [104]. This score established three different risk levels (low, medium, and high) based on four predictive components (recipient age, serum bilirubin, serum creatinine, and spell between premier and retransplantation). The 5-year survival was 68%, 62%, and 38% for low, intermediate and high risk, correspondingly. Concerns for this score still remained in recent years because it was developed before the MELD epoch, it does not investigate donor features and diverse recipients risk factors, and it is arithmetic complex [100]. The UCLA group [105] in 2011 developed a new risk stratification scoring that appoints one or two points for *preoperative clinical features* such as recipient age > 55 years, MELD >27, history of prior reLT, serum albumin <2.5 g/dL, interval of reLT within 15–180 days, necessity of ventilation before reLT, donor age > 45 years and *intraoperative features* like over-transfusion during reLT (>30 pRBC units). These points are added up to rank recipients into four risk categories (RC). Their 5-year survival was 79, 59, 49, and 22% for RS I, II,III, and IV, respectively, [100].

In general, retransplant in HCC recurrence after LT is not plausible (Recommendation in the **Table 11**), whereas various provided managements, such as LRT and systemic, have been employed, even in a compound manner, in an effort to extend survival [22].

Evaluation of HCC candidates to access LT	**Evidence Level**	**Strength of recommendation**
1. When considering treatment options for HCC patients, the BCLC staging system is the preferred staging system to assess the prognosis of patients with HCC	2b (P)	Strong
2. The TNM system (seventh edn), including pathological examination of the explanted liver, should be used for determining prognosis after transplantation with the addition of assessment of microvascular invasion.	2b (P)	Strong
3. Either dynamic CT or dynamic MRI with the presence of arterial enhancement followed by washout on portal venous or delayed imaging is the best noninvasive test to make a diagnosis in cirrhotic patients suspected of having HCC and for preoperative staging.	1b (D)	Strong
4. Extrahepatic staging should include CT of the chest and CT or MRI of the abdomen and pelvis.	3b (D)	Strong
5. Tumor biopsy is not required in cirrhotic patients considered for liver transplantation who have high-quality dynamic CT or MRI findings typical for HCC and a lesion larger than 1 cm according to current AASLD guidelines.	1b (D)	Weak
6. For patients with lesions smaller or equal to 10 mm, noninvasive imaging does not allow an accurate diagnosis and should not be used to make a decision for or against transplantation.	1b (D)	Strong
Criteria for listing candidates with HCC/liver cirrhosis for DDLT		
7. Liver transplantation should be reserved for HCC patients who have a predicted 5-year survival comparable to non-HCC patients.	NA	Weak
8. Preoperative assessment of the size of the largest tumor or total diameter of tumors should be the main consideration in selecting patients with HCC for liver transplantation.	2a (P)	Strong
9. The Milan criteria are currently the benchmark for the selection of HCC patients for liver transplantation, and the basis for comparison with other suggested criteria.	2a (P)	Strong
10. A modest expansion of the number of potential candidates may be considered on the basis of several studies showing comparable survival for patients outside the Milan criteria.	3b P)	Weak
11. Patients with worse prognoses may be considered for liver transplantation outside the Milan criteria if the dynamics of the waiting list allow it without undue prejudice to other recipients with a better prognosis.	NA	Weak
12. α-fetoprotein concentrations add prognostic information in HCC patients and may be used for making decisions regarding transplantation in combination with imaging criteria.	2b (P)	Weak
13. Biomarkers other than α-fetoprotein cannot yet be used for clinical decision-making regarding liver transplantation for HCC	2b (P)	Strong
14. Indication for liver transplantation in HCC should not rely on microvascular invasion because it cannot be reliably detected prior to transplantation.	2b (P)	Strong
Criteria for HCC candidates with non-cirrhotic livers		
15. The Milan criteria and its modifications are not applicable to patients with HCC developing in a non-cirrhotic liver. Such patients with non-resectable HCC and absence of macrovascular invasion and extrahepatic spread may be considered as appropriate candidates for liver transplantation.	4 (P)	Weak

Evaluation of HCC candidates to access LT	**Evidence Level**	**Strength of recommendation**
16. Patients with HCC in non-cirrhotic liver who were treated by resection, and have intrahepatic recurrence of HCC and no evidence of lymph node or macrovascular invasion, may be considered for salvage transplantation.	4 (P)	Weak
Role of downstaging		
17. Transplantation may be considered after successful downstaging.	5 (P)	Weak
18. Liver transplantation after successful downstaging should achieve a 5-year survival comparable to that of HCC patients who meet the criteria for liver transplantation without requiring downstaging.	5 (P)	Strong
19. Criteria for successful downstaging should include tumor size and number of viable tumors.	4 (P)	Strong
20. α-fetoprotein concentrations before and after downstaging may add additional information.	4 (P)	Weak
21. Based on existing evidence, no recommendation can be made for preferring a specific locoregional therapy for downstaging over others.	NA	None
Managing patients on the waiting list		
22. Periodic waiting-list monitoring should be performed by imaging (dynamic CT, dynamic MRI, or contrast-enhanced ultrasonography) and α-fetoprotein measurements.	5 (P)	Strong
23. Based on current absence of evidence, no recommendation can be made on bridging therapy in patients with UNOS T1 ($\leq$2 cm) HCC	NA	None
24. In patients with UNOS T2 (one nodule 2–5 cm or three or more nodules each $\leq$3 cm) HCC (Milan criteria) and a likely waiting time longer than 6 months, locoregional therapy may be appropriate.	4P	Weak
25. No recommendation can be made for preferring any type of locoregional therapy to others.	5 (P)	Strong
26. Patients found to have progressed beyond criteria acceptable for listing for liver transplantation should be placed on hold and considered for downstaging.	5 (P)	Strong
27. Patients with progressive disease in whom locoregional intervention is not considered appropriate, or is ineffective, should be removed from the waiting list.	5 (P)	Strong
Role of LDLT		
28. LDLT is acceptable for HCC patients who have an expected 5-year survival similar to comparably staged patients receiving a deceased-donor liver. In LDLT, careful attention should be given to psychosocial considerations regarding both donor and recipient	NA	Weak
29. LDLT must be restricted to centers of excellence in liver surgery and liver transplantation to minimize donor risk and maximize recipient outcome.	NA	Strong
30. In patients following LDLT for HCC within the accepted regional criteria for DDLT, retransplantation for graft failure is justified.	5 (P)	Weak
31. In patients following LDLT for HCC outside the accepted regional criteria for DDLT, retransplantation for graft failure using a deceased-donor organ is not recommended.	5 (P)	Strong
Posttransplant management		

Evaluation of HCC candidates to access LT	Evidence Level	Strength of recommendation
32. Post transplant monitoring may include 6–12 monthly contrast-enhanced CT or MRI imaging and α-fetoprotein measurements.	5 (P)	Weak
33. There is currently insufficient evidence from clinical trials to base a recommendation for choosing the type or dose of immunosuppression therapy to influence the incidence of HCC recurrence or its prognosis.	NA	None
34. Based on current evidence, no recommendation can be made on the use of mTOR inhibitors solely to reduce the risk of HCC recurrence outside clinical trials.	NA	None
35. The current evidence does not justify the routine use of adjuvant antitumor therapy after liver transplantation for HCC outside of a controlled clinical trial.	NA	Weak
36. HCC recurrence after liver transplantation may be treated by surgery for resectable lesions or by locoregional therapy or systemic therapy (including sorafenib) for unresectable lesions.	4 (P)	Weak
37. Liver retransplantation is not appropriate treatment for recurrent HCC.	NA	Strong

Level of evidence for each recommendation refers to the Oxford classification. P = prognosis. D = diagnosis. NA = not applicable.

Table 11.
Recommendations for liver transplantation for HCC: An international consensus conference report in 2010 [44].

8. Contraindications of liver transplantation in the HCC patients

Contraindications of LT comprise *clinical* and *psychosocial* reasons and could be further defined as *liver* and *non-liver relative* and *absolute* contraindications. *Clinically* major factors to preclude surgery as severe cardio-pulmonary disorders, ongoing sepsis, widespread portal and visceral venous thrombosis, and progressed or metastatic cancer. *Relative* contraindications differ between centers and include advanced age or acquired immune deficiency syndrome (AIDS), but this may be individualized considered. *Psychosocial contraindications* comprise inadequate or without social assistance, unstable psychiatric disorder, ongoing addiction, or limited insurance for post-LT medicaments [106]. Outcomes of LT for HCC can considerably differ between patients with the same morphologic HCC registration criteria; thus, plenty of these contraindications are relative or transitory instead of absolute.

Metastasis out of liver is generally considered an obvious *contraindication* for LT [6]. To most Western centers, portal vein or hepatic veins macroscopic invasion are *absolute contraindications* for LT, considering it is the most important and independent risk factor for posttransplant HCC recurrence, and thus for critical diminution in survival [107].

In the US, current UNOS organ distribution strategy [108] defines the following cases to be contraindications to LT and/or will not be provided MELD exception for HCC [5]:

- Main portal or hepatic veins macroscopic invasion;
- Extrahepatic tumor spread;
- Fractured HCC;
- Early stage (T1): Resection feasible (solitary tumor <2 cm);

- History of HCC steadily cured >2 years ago without recurrence;
- Tumor number and size advancement despite LRT; or those who were exceeding conventional inclusion criteria;
- Serum AFP consistently >1000 ng/mL and unable to go down below 500.

Similarly in France and Canada, the AFP level ≥ 1000 ng/dL is disqualified to access for DDLT [35, 65].

9. Current recommendations for liver transplantation for HCC

9.1 International consensus conference report in 2010

Though LT is an extensively recognized treatment modality for HCC, arguments still persist and no single guideline was universally approved. An international agreement assembly in Swiss (2010), revised recent practices regarding liver transplantation in HCC and to build globally acknowledged declarations and guidance (**Table 11**) [44].

Recommendations.

- LT is recommended as the first-line option for HCC within Milan criteria but unfit to liver resection (*evidence high*; *recommendation strong*). Milan criteria are the benchmark for the selection of patients with HCC for LT and the basis for comparison with other suggested criteria.
- Agreements on extended criteria for LT in HCC have not been achieved. Patients exceeding Milan criteria can be considered for LT after successful downstaging to fulfill these criteria, within defined protocols (*evidence moderate*; *recommendation weak*).
- Combination criteria that consider surrogates of tumor biology (AFP) and response to neoadjuvant treatments (bridging or downstaging tumors) together with tumor burden are likely to replace conventional criteria to access LT. Combined criteria should be investigated and determined a priori, validated prospectively, and auditable at any time (*evidence low*; *recommendation strong*).
- Tumor vascular invasion and extrahepatic metastases are absolute contraindications for LT in HCC (*evidence high*).
- There is no contraindication to use marginal cadaveric grafts for LT in HCC patients (evidence moderate). Prioritizing a cadaveric graft allocation, for patients with or without HCC, within a common waiting list, is complex, and no system can serve all regions. Prioritization criteria for HCC should at least include tumor burden, tumor biology indicators, waiting time, and response to tumor treatment (*evidence moderate*; *recommendation strong*).
- Transplant benefit may need to be considered alongside the conventional transplant principles of urgency and utility in decision-making, regarding patient selection and prioritization, depending on list composition and dynamics (evidence moderate; recommendation weak).
- In LT candidates with HCC, the use of pre-transplant (neoadjuvant) LRT is recommended if feasible as it reduces the risk of pre-LT dropout and aims at reducing post-LT recurrence, particularly when complete or partial tumor response is achieved (*evidence low*; *recommendation strong*).
- Although the contribution of living donation to LT for HCC in Europe is still marginal, living donor LT for HCC remains an option to be explored in selected patients and in experienced centers, according to waiting list time and dynamics, and within donor-recipient double equipoise principles (*evidence low*).

Table 12.
EASL clinical practice guidelines recommendations (2018) [6].

9.2 EASL clinical practice guidelines recommendations (2018)

The clinical practice guidelines will be extracted here its recent (2018) advice for the clinical management, particularly relevant to LT for HCC (**Table 12**).

9.3 The UNOS 2022 recommendation: Adult MELD exceptions for HCC

LT candidate receives a MELD or a PELD score (if age < 12) for organ distribution. This score reflects the patient's illness severity by 3-month mortality risk without LT. When the formal score does not express the candidate's actual medical urgency, their LT program may need an exception score. A candidate fulfills criteria for one of nine diagnoses in policy is permitted for a standardized MELD exception. If the candidate unfits criteria for standardized exception, Review Board should study this request (**Table 13**) [108].

10. Ethical considerations in LT for HCC

The main issue in LDLT is donor safety because of the risk of complications or death, even if small. Currently, the reported morbidity and mortality of living donor hepatectomy is 16 and 0.2%, respectively [109]. The concept of "*double equipoise*" was proposed to describe the balance between the recipient's survival benefit with LDLT and the risk of a complication or death of a healthy donor [44]. LDLT for patients with HCC is still controversial with the ethical dilemma to risk a healthy person for a recipient that has a fatal disease with a high risk of recurrence.

Principle	Application and considerations
Autonomy	Does the donor have enough information regarding the circumstances of living donation to provide adequate informed consent? Is there "right to donate"? Considerations of donor's actual motivation for undertaking an LDLT?
Nonmaleficence	How do transplant teams respect the principle of "*do no harm*" knowing that living donors assume medical risk without any direct medical benefit? How can transplant teams minimize donor risks, with medical and psychosocial complications? [110]
Utility	Assigned to optimization of posttransplant results. Concentrated on posttransplant prognosis with intention to diminish HCC recurrence and extending survival [22]. Despite donor pool improval, should LDLT be inspired, even likely not comparable recipient results?
Urgency	Diminish mortality risk before LT. Typically devoted to non-HCC/cirrhotic patients, with worse short-term outcomes while on the waiting list because of a rapid deterioration of liver function. It is ethical enigma; donated organs are distributed to the "*sickest patient first*" among non-cancer candidates, but to the "*earliest patient first*" among HCC candidates for LT, irrespective of their survival prospects with other treatment modalities.
Beneficence	Rating patients with the pure survival benefit and optimization survival gain after LT. Necessity for policy adjustments so as to preclude vain LT or give prioritization to higher risk of recurrence patients.
Equity	Should "social worth" criteria have incorporated into the organ allocation system, hence demanding LDLT consideration?

Table 13.
Application and considering principles of medical ethics in LDLT settings [22, 110].

With obvious benefit of DDLT, LDLT presents ethical challenges as to respect principles of medical ethics, including autonomy, nonmaleficence, beneficence.

11. Conclusions and future directions

Liver malignancies (with HCC in >97% of cases) have become the main indications (40–60%) of liver transplantation (LT) over the last decades.

Anticipation of outcomes in LT for HCC continues to be a challenge. A practical staging system for HCC which is also a powerful predictor for recurrent after LT is yet to be reached with universally acceptance. Tumor biology characters by AFP and PIVKA-II (DCP) should be put on top of tumor morphology.

LT indications for HCC, initially relied on static staging, have converted to a dynamic process comprising treatment-response and tumor biology and should focus on candidates with predicted recurrent-free rate of >70% as with non-HCC patients. This will enable more candidates exceeding MC to access LT while securing their acceptable outcomes.

Inclusion criteria for LT in HCC patients differ between centers and regions. With justified selection, liver transplantation would be a potential management to cure the liver cancer patient, especially in the setting of underlying liver cirrhosis.

LDLT is really an excellent and effective alternative in regions with scarce of deceased-donor organs. Together with ethical issues and the "*double equipoise*" concept, much consideration should be raised on how far we can expand the LT indication for HCC patients. Especially in the scenario of failure of primary LT on a far advanced HCC patient that requires a retransplant sharing the same donor pool of DDLT as it could obviously negatively impact another candidate that should have received that organ.

Acknowledgements

Thanks to Professor Kim Jong Man (Dept of Surgery, SMC, Sungkyunkwan University School of Medicine, Seoul, Korea) for his kind mentorship and sharing the copyright of material using in this chapter.

Author details

Nam Hoang Duc
General Surgery Department, Hue Central Hospital, Hue City, Vietnam

*Address all correspondence to: hoangducnammd@gmail.com

References

[1] World Health Organization. Global cancer observatory. Available from: https://gco.iarc.fr/. 2022. [Accessed: December 20, 2022]

[2] Ziogas IA, Tsoulfas G. The evolution of criteria for liver transplantation for hepatocellular carcinoma: From Milan to San Francisco and all around the world ! Revista de la Facultad de Medicina Humana. 2017;**17**(3):56-69

[3] Arslanoglu A, Seyal AR, Sodagari F, Sahin A, Miller FH, Salem R, et al. Current guidelines for the diagnosis and Management of Hepatocellular Carcinoma: A comparative review. AJR. American Journal of Roentgenology. 2016;**207**(5):W88-W98. DOI: 10.2214/AJR.15.15490. Epub 2016 Aug 4

[4] Maggs JRL, Suddle AR, Aluvihare V, Heneghan MA. Systematic review: The role of liver transplantation in the management of hepatocellular carcinoma. Alimentary Pharmacology & Therapeutics. 2012;**35**:1113-1134

[5] Terrault NA, Francoz C, Berenguer M, Charlton M, Heimbach J. Liver transplantation 2023: Status report, current and future challenges. Clinical Gastroenterology and Hepatology: The Official Clinical Practice Journal of the American Gastroenterological Association. 2023;**21**(8):2150-2166. DOI: 10.1016/j.cgh.2023.04.005

[6] EASL Clinical Practice Guidelines. Management of hepatocellular carcinoma. Journal of Hepatology. 2018;**69**(1):182-236

[7] Mahmud N. Selection for liver transplantation: Indications and evaluation. Current Hepatology Reports. 2020;**19**:203-212

[8] Mazzaferro V, Regalia E, Doci R, Andreola S, Pulvirenti A, Bozzetti F, et al. Liver transplantation for the treatment of small hepatocellular carcinomas in patients with cirrhosis. The New England Journal of Medicine. 1996;**334**:693-699

[9] Duvoux C, Lerut JP. Selection criteria and outcome of liver transplantation for neoplastic liver diseases. In: Burra P, editor. Textbook of Liver Transplantation. Springer: Cham; 2022. pp. 55-72

[10] Todo S, Furukawa H, Tada M, Japanese Liver Transplantation Study Group. Extending indication: Role of living donor liver transplantation for hepatocellular carcinoma. Liver Transplantation. 2007;**13**(11 Suppl. 2):S48-S54

[11] Vauthey JN, Dixon E, Abdalla EK, et al. Pretreatment assessment of hepatocellular carcinoma: Expert consensus statement. HPB: The Official Journal of the International Hepato Pancreato Biliary Association. 2010;**12**(5):289-299

[12] Yao FY, Xiao L, Bass NM, Kerlan R, Ascher NL, Roberts JP. Liver transplantation for hepatocellular carcinoma: Validation of the UCSF-expanded criteria based on preoperative imaging. American Journal of Transplantation. 2007;**7**(11):2587-2596. DOI: 10.1111/j.1600-6143.2007.01965.x

[13] Reig M, Forner A, Rimola J, et al. BCLC strategy for prognosis prediction and treatment recommendation: The 2022 update. Journal of Hepatology. 2022;**76**(3):681-693

[14] Yao FY, Ferrell L, Bass NM, Watson JJ, Bacchetti P, Venook A, et al. Liver transplantation for hepatocellular carcinoma: Expansion of the tumor size

limits does not adversely impact survival. Hepatology. 2001;**33**:1394-1403

[15] Onaca N, Stone MJ, Fulmer JM, Klintmalm. Transplantation for primary hepatic malignancy. In: Busuttil RW, Klintmalm GBG, editors. Transplantation of the Liver. 3rd ed. Philadelphia: Elsevier Saunders; 2015. pp. 189-204

[16] Rich NE, Parikh ND, Singal AG. Hepatocellular carcinoma and liver transplantation: Changing patterns and practices. Current Treatment Options in Gastroenterology. 2017;**15**:296-304. DOI: 10.1007/s11938-017-0133-3

[17] Singal AK, Kamath PS. Management of the patient on the waiting list, scoring systems, and priority. In: Burra P, editor. Textbook of Liver Transplantation. Springer: Cham; 2022. pp. 121-132

[18] Halazun KJ, Patzer RE, Rana AA, et al. Standing the test of time: Outcomes of a decade of prioritizing patients with hepatocellular carcinoma, results of the UNOS natural geographic experiment. Hepatology. 2014;**60**(6):1957-1962

[19] Ishaque T, Massie AB, Bowring MG, et al. Liver transplantation and waitlist mortality for HCC and non-HCC candidates following the 2015 HCC exception policy change. American Journal of Transplantation. 2019;**19**(2):564-572

[20] Heimbach JK. Evolution of liver transplant selection criteria and U.S. allocation policy for patients with hepatocellular carcinoma. Seminars in Liver Disease. 2020;**40**:358-364

[21] Azzam AZ. Liver transplantation as a management of hepatocellular carcinoma. World Journal of Hepatology. 2015;7(10):1347-1354

[22] Bhoori S, Mazzaferro V. Current challenges in liver transplantation for hepatocellular carcinoma [published correction appears in best Pract res Clin Gastroenterol. 2014 Dec;28(6):1115-6]. Best Practice & Research. Clinical Gastroenterology. 2014;**28**(5):867-879. DOI: 10.1016/j.bpg.2014.08.001

[23] Kim SJ, Kim JM. Prediction models of hepatocellular carcinoma recurrence after liver transplantation: A comprehensive review. Clinical and Molecular Hepatology. 2022;**28**(4):739-753

[24] Bismuth H, Chiche L, Adam R, Castaing D, Diamond T, Dennison A. Liver resection versus transplantation for hepatocellular carcinoma in cirrhotic patients. Annals of Surgery. 1993;**218**:145-151

[25] Herrero JI, Sangro B, Quiroga J, Pardo F, Herraiz M, Cienfuegos JA, et al. Influence of tumor characteristics on the outcome of liver transplantation among patients with liver cirrhosis and hepatocellular carcinoma. Liver Transplantation: Official Publication of the American Association for the Study of Liver Diseases and the International Liver Transplantation Society. 2001;**7**:631-636. DOI: 10.1053/jlts.2001.25458

[26] Roayaie S, Frischer JS, Emre SH, et al. Long-term results with multimodal adjuvant therapy and liver transplantation for the treatment of hepatocellular carcinomas larger than 5 centimeters. Annals of Surgery. 2002;**235**(4):533-539. DOI: 10.1097/00000658-200204000-00012

[27] Kneteman NM, Oberholzer J, Saghier MA, et al. Sirolimus-based immunosuppression for liver transplantation in the presence of extended criteria for hepatocellular carcinoma. Liver Transplantation. 2004;**10**(10):1301-1311. DOI: 10.1002/lt.20237

[28] Onaca N, Davis GL, Goldstein RM, Jennings LW, Klintmalm GB. Expanded

criteria for liver transplantation in patients with hepatocellular carcinoma: A report from the international registry of hepatic Tumors in liver transplantation. Liver Transplantation. 2007;**13**(3):391-399

[29] Zheng SS, Xu X, Wu J, et al. Liver transplantation for hepatocellular carcinoma: Hangzhou experiences [retracted in: Transplantation. 2019 Aug;103(8):1736]. Transplantation. 2008;**85**(12):1726-1732

[30] Silva M, Moya A, Berenguer M, et al. Expanded criteria for liver transplantation in patients with cirrhosis and hepatocellular carcinoma. Liver Transplantation. 2008;**14**(10):1449-1460

[31] Mazzaferro V, Llovet JM, Miceli R, et al. Predicting survival after liver transplantation in patients with hepatocellular carcinoma beyond the Milan criteria: A retrospective, exploratory analysis. The Lancet Oncology. 2009;**10**(1):35-43. DOI: 10.1016/S1470-2045(08)70284-5

[32] Toso C, Asthana S, Bigam DL, Shapiro AM, Kneteman NM. Reassessing selection criteria prior to liver transplantation for hepatocellular carcinoma utilizing the scientific registry of transplant recipients database. Hepatology. 2009;**49**(3):832-838. DOI: 10.1002/hep.22693

[33] Lai Q, Avolio AW, Graziadei I, Otto G, Rossi M, Tisone G, et al. Alpha-fetoprotein and modified response evaluation criteria in solid tumors progression after locoregional therapy as predictors of hepatocellular cancer recurrence and death after transplantation. Liver Transplantation. 2013;**19**(10):1108-1118

[34] DuBay D, Sandroussi C, Sandhu L, et al. Liver transplantation for advanced hepatocellular carcinoma using poor tumor differentiation on biopsy as an exclusion criterion. Annals of Surgery. 2011;**253**(1):166-172

[35] Duvoux C, Roudot-Thoraval F, Decaens T, et al. Liver transplantation for hepatocellular carcinoma: A model including alpha-fetoprotein improves the performance of Milan criteria. Gastroenterology. 2012;**143**:986-994, e3. quiz e14–e15

[36] Grąt M, Kornasiewicz O, Lewandowski Z, et al. Combination of morphologic criteria and α-fetoprotein in selection of patients with hepatocellular carcinoma for liver transplantation minimizes the problem of posttransplant tumor recurrence. World Journal of Surgery. 2014;**38**(10):2698-2707

[37] Mehta N, Heimbach J, Harnois DM, et al. Validation of a risk estimation of tumor recurrence after transplant (RETREAT) score for hepatocellular carcinoma recurrence after liver transplant. JAMA Oncology. 2017;**3**(4):493-500. DOI: 10.1001/jamaoncol.2016.5116

[38] Mehta N, Dodge JL, Roberts JP, Yao FY. Validation of the prognostic power of the RETREAT score for hepatocellular carcinoma recurrence using the UNOS database. American Journal of Transplantation. 2018;**18**(5):1206-1213. DOI: 10.1111/ajt.14549

[39] Halazun KJ, Najjar M, Abdelmessih RM, et al. Recurrence after liver transplantation for hepatocellular carcinoma: A new moral to the story. Annals of Surgery. 2017;**265**(3):557-564

[40] Mazzaferro V, Sposito C, Zhou J, Pinna AD, De Carlis L, Fan J, et al. Metroticket 2.0 model for analysis of competing risks of death after liver transplantation for hepatocellular carcinoma. Gastroenterology. 2018;**154**:128-139

[41] Goldberg D, Mantero A, Newcomb C, Delgado C, Forde KA, Kaplan DE, et al. Predicting survival after liver transplantation in patients with hepatocellular carcinoma using the LiTES-HCC score. Journal of Hepatology. 2021;**74**:1398-1406

[42] Bismuth H, Majno PE, Adam R. Liver transplantation for hepatocellular carcinoma. Seminars in Liver Disease. 1999;**19**:311-322. DOI: 10.1055/s-2007-1007120

[43] Pavel MC, Fuster J. Expansion of the hepatocellular carcinoma Milan criteria in liver transplantation: Future directions. World Journal of Gastroenterology. 2018;**24**(32):3626-3636

[44] Clavien PA, Lesurtel M, Bossuyt PM, et al. Recommendations for liver transplantation for hepatocellular carcinoma: An international consensus conference report. The Lancet Oncology. 2012;**13**(1):e11-e22

[45] Sugawara Y, Tamura S, Makuuchi M. Living donor liver transplantation for hepatocellular carcinoma: Tokyo university series. Digestive Diseases. 2007;**25**(4):310-312. DOI: 10.1159/000106910

[46] Lee SG, Hwang S, Moon DB, et al. Expanded indication criteria of living donor liver transplantation for hepatocellular carcinoma at one large-volume center. Liver Transplantation. 2008;**14**(7):935-945

[47] Soejima Y, Taketomi A, Yoshizumi T, et al. Extended indication for living donor liver transplantation in patients with hepatocellular carcinoma. Transplantation. 2007;**83**(7):893-899

[48] Chan SC, Fan ST, Lo CM, et al. A decade of right liver adult-to-adult living donor liver transplantation: The recipient mid-term outcomes. Annals of Surgery. 2008;**248**(3):411-419

[49] Concejero A, Chen CL, Wang CC, et al. Living donor liver transplantation for hepatocellular carcinoma: A single-center experience in Taiwan. Transplantation. 2008;**85**(3):398-406

[50] Taketomi A, Sanefuji K, Soejima Y, et al. Impact of des-gamma-carboxy prothrombin and tumor size on the recurrence of hepatocellular carcinoma after living donor liver transplantation. Transplantation. 2009;**87**(4):531-537. DOI: 10.1097/TP.0b013e3181943bee

[51] Ito T, Takada Y, Ueda M, Haga H, Maetani Y, Oike F, et al. Expansion of selection criteria for patients with hepatocellular carcinoma in living donor liver transplantation. Liver Transplantation. 2007;**13**:1637-1644

[52] Furukawa H, Shimamura T, Suzuki T, et al. Liver transplantation for hepatocellular carcinoma: The Japanese experience. Journal of Hepato-Biliary-Pancreatic Sciences. 2010;**17**:533-538

[53] Yang K, Lee TB, Choi BH, Park YM, Ryu JH, Joo DJ, et al. Development and applicability of the A-P 200 criteria for liver transplantation for hepatocellular carcinoma. Transplantation Proceedings. 2016;**48**(10):3317-3322. DOI: 10.1016/j.transproceed.2016.08.050

[54] Kaido T, Mori A, Ogura Y, et al. Living donor liver transplantation for recurrent hepatocellular carcinoma after liver resection. Surgery. 2012;**151**(1):55-60. DOI: 10.1016/j.surg.2011.06.032

[55] Kim JM, Kwon CH, Joh JW, et al. Expanded criteria for liver transplantation in patients with hepatocellular carcinoma. Transplantation Proceedings. 2014;**46**(3):726-729

[56] Hong G, Suh KS, Suh SW, et al. Alpha-fetoprotein and (18)F-FDG positron emission tomography predict tumor recurrence better than Milan criteria in living donor liver transplantation. Journal

of Hepatology. 2016;**64**(4):852-859. DOI: 10.1016/j.jhep.2015.11.033

[57] Lee JH, Cho Y, Kim HY, et al. Serum tumor markers provide refined prognostication in selecting liver transplantation candidate for hepatocellular carcinoma patients beyond the Milan criteria. Annals of Surgery. 2016;**263**(5):842-850. DOI: 10.1097/SLA.0000000000001578

[58] Lee EC, Kim SH, Shim JR, Park SJ. Small-for-size grafts increase recurrence of hepatocellular carcinoma in liver transplantation beyond Milan criteria. Liver Transplantation. 2018;**24**(1):35-43

[59] Shimamura T, Akamatsu N, Fujiyoshi M, et al. Expanded living-donor liver transplantation criteria for patients with hepatocellular carcinoma based on the Japanese nationwide survey: The 5-5-500 rule - A retrospective study. Transplant International. 2019;**32**(4):356-368

[60] Vibert E, Azoulay D, Hoti E, Iacopinelli S, Samuel D, Salloum C, et al. Progression of alphafetoprotein before liver transplantation for hepatocellular carcinoma in cirrhotic patients: A critical factor. American Journal of Transplantation. 2010;**10**:129-137

[61] Notarpaolo A, Layese R, Magistri P, Gambato M, Colledan M, Magini G, et al. Validation of the AFP model as a predictor of HCC recurrence in patients with viral hepatitis-related cirrhosis who had received a liver transplant for HCC. Journal of Hepatology. 2017;**66**(3):552-559

[62] Varona MA, Soriano A, Aguirre-Jaime A, Garrido S, Oton E, Diaz D, et al. Risk factors of hepatocellular carcinoma recurrence after liver transplantation: Accuracy of the alpha-fetoprotein model in a single-center experience. Transplantation Proceedings. 2015;**47**(1):84-89

[63] Piñero F, Tisi Baña M, de Ataide EC, Hoyos Duque S, Marciano S, Varón A, et al. Liver transplantation for hepatocellular carcinoma: Evaluation of the alpha-fetoprotein model in a multicenter cohort from Latin America. Liver International. 2016;**36**(11):1657-1667

[64] Cillo U, Vitale A, Bassanello M, et al. Liver transplantation for the treatment of moderately or well-differentiated hepatocellular carcinoma. Annals of Surgery. 2004;**239**(2):150-159

[65] Sapisochin G, Goldaracena N, Laurence JM, et al. The extended Toronto criteria for liver transplantation in patients with hepatocellular carcinoma: A prospective validation study. Hepatology. 2016;**64**:2077-2088

[66] Decaens T, Roudot-Thoraval F, Badran H, et al. Impact of tumour differentiation to select patients before liver transplantation for hepatocellular carcinoma. Liver International. 2011;**31**(6):792-801

[67] Lin C-C, Elsarawy AMAA, Chen C-L. Living Donor Liver Transplantation for Hepatocellular Carcinoma. London, UK: InTechOpen; 2017. DOI: 10.5772/65109

[68] Hsu C-C, Chen C-L, Wang C-C, Lin C-C, Yong C-C, Wang S-H, et al. Combination of FDG-PET and UCSF criteria for predicting HCC recurrence after living donor liver transplantation. Transplantation. 2016;**100**(9):1925-1932

[69] Chalaye J, Costentin CE, Luciani A, et al. Positron emission tomography/computed tomography with 18F-fluorocholine improve tumor staging and treatment allocation in patients with hepatocellular carcinoma. Journal of Hepatology. 2018;**69**(2):336-344

[70] Meischl T, Rasoul-Rockenschaub S, Györi G, et al. C-reactive protein

is an independent predictor for hepatocellular carcinoma recurrence after liver transplantation. PLoS One. 2019;**14**(5):e0216677. DOI: 10.1371/journal.pone.0216677 [Accessed: May 29, 2019]

[71] Kornberg A, Witt U, Schernhammer M, et al. The role of preoperative albumin-bilirubin grade for oncological risk stratification in liver transplant patients with hepatocellular carcinoma. Journal of Surgical Oncology. 2019;**120**(7):1126-1136. DOI: 10.1002/jso.25721

[72] Firl DJ, Sasaki K, Agopian VG, et al. Charting the path forward for risk prediction in liver transplant for hepatocellular carcinoma: International validation of HALTHCC among 4,089 patients. Hepatology. 2020;**71**(2):569-582. DOI: 10.1002/hep.30838

[73] Aloia TA, Adam R, Samuel D, Azoulay D, Castaing D. A decision analysis model identifies the interval of efficacy for transarterial chemoembolization (TACE) in cirrhotic patients with hepatocellular carcinoma awaiting liver transplantation. Journal of Gastrointestinal Surgery. 2007;**11**:1328-1332

[74] Kollmann D, Selzner N, Selzner M. Bridging to liver transplantation in HCC patients. Langenbeck's Archives of Surgery. 2017 Sep;**402**(6):863-871. DOI: 10.1007/s00423-017-1609-2

[75] Lai Q, Avolio AW, Manzia TM, Sorge R, Agnes S, Tisone G, et al. Combination of biological and morphological parameters for the selection of patients with hepatocellular carcinoma waiting for liver transplantation. Clinical Transplantation. 2012;**26**(2):E125-E131

[76] Yao FY, Mehta N, Flemming J, et al. Downstaging of hepatocellular cancer before liver transplant: Long-term outcome compared to tumors within Milan criteria. Hepatology. 2015;**61**(6):1968-1977

[77] Mehta N. Liver transplantation criteria for hepatocellular carcinoma, including Posttransplant management. Clinics in Liver Disease. 2021;**17**(5):332-336. Published 2021 Jun 4. DOI: 10.1002/cld.1054

[78] Ravaioli M, Grazi GL, Piscaglia F, et al. Liver transplantation for hepatocellular carcinoma: Results of down-staging in patients initially outside the Milan selection criteria. American Journal of Transplantation. 2008;**8**(12):2547-2557

[79] Lai Q, Nicolini D, Inostroza Nunez M, et al. A novel prognostic index in patients with hepatocellular cancer waiting for liver transplantation: Time-radiological-response-alpha-fetoprotein-INflammation (TRAIN) score. Annals of Surgery. 2016;**264**(5):787-796

[80] Mazzaferro V, Citterio D, Bhoori S, et al. Liver transplantation in hepatocellular carcinoma after tumour downstaging (XXL): A randomised, controlled, phase 2b/3 trial [published correction appears in lancet Oncol. 2020 Aug;21(8):e373]. The Lancet Oncology. 2020;**21**(7):947-956

[81] Heimbach JK, Kulik LM, Finn RS, et al. AASLD guidelines for the treatment of hepatocellular carcinoma. Hepatology. 2018;**67**(1):358-380. DOI: 10.1002/hep.29086

[82] Graziadei IW, Sandmueller H, Waldenberger P, Koenigsrainer A, Nachbaur K, Jaschke W, et al. Chemoembolization followed by liver transplantation for hepatocellular carcinoma impedes tumor progression while on the waiting list and leads to excellent outcome. Liver

Transplantation. 2003;**9**:557-563. DOI: 10.1053/jlts.2003.50106

[83] Otto G, Herber S, Heise M, et al. Response to transarterial chemoembolization as a biological selection criterion for liver transplantation in hepatocellular carcinoma. Liver Transplantation. 2006;**12**(8):1260-1267. DOI: 10.1002/lt.20837

[84] Millonig G, Graziadei IW, Freund MC, Jaschke W, Stadlmann S, Ladurner R, et al. Response to preoperative chemoembolization correlates with outcome after liver transplantation in patients with hepatocellular carcinoma. Liver Transplantation. 2007;**13**:272-279

[85] Chapman WC, Majella Doyle MB, Stuart JE, et al. Outcomes of neoadjuvant transarterial chemoembolization to downstage hepatocellular carcinoma before liver transplantation. Annals of Surgery. 2008;**248**(4):617-625

[86] Lewandowski RJ, Kulik LM, Riaz A, et al. A comparative analysis of transarterial downstaging for hepatocellular carcinoma: Chemoembolization versus radioembolization. American Journal of Transplantation. 2009;**9**(8):1920-1928

[87] De Luna W, Sze DY, Ahmed A, et al. Transarterial chemoinfusion for hepatocellular carcinoma as downstaging therapy and a bridge toward liver transplantation. American Journal of Transplantation. 2009;**9**(5):1158-1168

[88] Jang JW, You CR, Kim CW, et al. Benefit of downsizing hepatocellular carcinoma in a liver transplant population. Alimentary Pharmacology & Therapeutics. 2010;**31**(3):415-423. DOI: 10.1111/j.1365-2036.2009.04167.x

[89] Pommergaard HC, Rostved AA, Adam R, et al. Locoregional treatments before liver transplantation for hepatocellular carcinoma: A study from the European liver transplant registry. Transplant International. 2018;**31**(5):531-539. DOI: 10.1111/tri.13123

[90] Ogawa K, Kaido T, Okajima H, et al. Impact of pretreatments on outcomes after living donor liver transplantation for hepatocellular carcinoma. Journal of Hepato-Biliary-Pancreatic Sciences. 2019;**26**(2):73-81

[91] Mehta N, Dodge JL, Roberts JP, Hirose R, Yao FY. Alpha-fetoprotein decrease from > 1,000 to < 500 ng/mL in patients with hepatocellular carcinoma leads to improved Posttransplant outcomes. Hepatology. 2019;**69**(3):1193-1205

[92] Sinha J, Mehta N, Dodge JL, Poltavskiy E, Roberts J, Yao F. Are there upper limits in tumor burden for down-staging of hepatocellular carcinoma to liver transplant? Analysis of the all-comers protocol. Hepatology. 2019;**70**(4):1185-1196

[93] Vutien P, Dodge J, Bambha KM, et al. A simple measure of hepatocellular carcinoma burden predicts tumor recurrence after liver transplantation: The recurrent hepatocellular carcinoma-initial, maximum, last classification. Liver Transplantation. 2019;**25**(4):559-570

[94] DiNorcia J, Florman SS, Haydel B, et al. Pathologic response to Pretransplant Locoregional therapy is predictive of patient outcome after liver transplantation for hepatocellular carcinoma: Analysis from the US Multicenter HCC transplant consortium. Annals of Surgery. 2020;**271**(4):616-624

[95] Fisher RA, Kulik LM, Freise CE, Lok AS, Shearon TH, Brown RS Jr, et al. Hepatocellular carcinoma recurrence and death following living and deceased donor liver transplantation. American Journal of Transplantation. 2007;**7**(6):1601-1608

[96] Liang W, Wu L, Ling X, et al. Living donor liver transplantation versus deceased donor liver transplantation for hepatocellular carcinoma: A meta-analysis. Liver Transplantation. 2012;**18**(10):1226-1236. DOI: 10.1002/lt.23490

[97] Cauley RP, Potanos K, Fullington N, et al. The effect of graft type on mortality in liver transplantation for hepatocellular carcinoma. Annals of Transplantation. 2015;**20**:175-185. Published 2015 Mar 30. DOI: 10.12659/AOT.892613

[98] Kim KH, Park JI. Living-related liver transplantation. In: Burra P, editor. Textbook of Liver Transplantation. Vol. 2022. Switzerland AG: Springer, Champions; 2022. pp. 203-218

[99] Lee HW, Suh KS. Expansion of the criteria for living donor liver transplantation for hepatocellular carcinoma. Current Opinion in Organ Transplantation. 2016;**21**(2):231-237

[100] Cillo U, Bertacco A. Liver Retransplantation. In: Burra P, editor. Textbook of Liver Transplantation. Cham: Springer; 2022. DOI: 10.1007/978-3-030-82930-8_24

[101] Adam R, Karam V, Delvart V, O'Grady J, Mirza D, Klempnauer J, et al. Evolution of indications and results of liver transplantation in Europe. A report from the European liver transplant registry (ELTR). Journal of Hepatology. 2012;**57**:675-688

[102] Kim HJ, Larson JJ, Lim YS, et al. Impact of MELD on waitlist outcome of retransplant candidates. American Journal of Transplantation. 2010;**10**(12):2652-2657

[103] Biggins SW, Gralla J, Dodge JL, et al. Survival benefit of repeat liver transplantation in the United States: A serial MELD analysis by hepatitis C status and donor risk index. American Journal of Transplantation. 2014;**14**(11):2588-2594. DOI: 10.1111/ajt.12867

[104] Rosen HR, Prieto M, Casanovas-Taltavull T, et al. Validation and refinement of survival models for liver retransplantation. Hepatology. 2003;**38**(2):460-469

[105] Hong JC, Kaldas FM, Kositamongkol P, et al. Predictive index for long-term survival after retransplantation of the liver in adult recipients: Analysis of a 26-year experience in a single center. Annals of Surgery. 2011;**254**(3):444-448; discussion 448-9

[106] Pomposelli JJ, Simpson MA, Simon C, Pomfret EA. Liver transplantation. In: JLR F, editor. Transplantation. 5th ed. New York, Oxford: Saunders Elsevier; 2014. pp. 127-148

[107] Andreou A, Bahra M, Schmelzle M, Öllinger R, Sucher R, Sauer IM, et al. Predictive factors for extrahepatic recurrence of hepatocellular carcinoma following liver transplantation. Clinical Transplantation. 2016;**30**:819-827

[108] Organ Procurement and Transplantation Network. UNOS Organ Allocation policy. 2023. Available from: https://optn.transplant. hrsa.gov/media/2846/liver_guidance_hcc_201706.pdf. [Accessed: December 28, 2022]

[109] Ince V, Sahin TT, Akbulut S, Yilmaz S. Liver transplantation for hepatocellular carcinoma: Historical evolution of transplantation criteria. World Journal of Clinical Cases. 2022;**10**(29):10413-10427

[110] Nizamuddin I, Gordon EJ, Levitsky J. Ethical issues when considering liver donor versus deceased donor liver transplantation. Clinical Liver Disease (Hoboken). 2021;**17**(2):71-74. DOI: 10.1002/cld.982 [Accessed: February 28, 2021]